Wellbeing and Resilience for Nursing, Health and Social Care Students

Wellbeing and Resilience for Nursing, Health and Social Care Students

Annette Chowthi-Williams

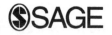

Los Angeles | London | New Delhi
Singapore | Washington DC | Melbourne

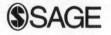

Los Angeles | London | New Delhi
Singapore | Washington DC | Melbourne

SAGE Publications Ltd
1 Oliver's Yard
55 City Road
London EC1Y 1SP

SAGE Publications Inc.
2455 Teller Road
Thousand Oaks, California 91320

SAGE Publications India Pvt Ltd
B 1/I 1 Mohan Cooperative Industrial Area
Mathura Road
New Delhi 110 044

SAGE Publications Asia-Pacific Pte Ltd
3 Church Street
#10-04 Samsung Hub
Singapore 049483

Editor: Laura Walmsley
Editorial assistant: Sahar Jamfar
Production editor: Victoria Nicholas
Marketing manager: Ruslana Khatagova
Cover design: Wendy Scott
Typeset by: TNQ Technologies

Library of Congress Control Number: 2022942654

British Library Cataloguing in Publication data

A catalogue record for this book is available from the British Library

ISBN 978-1-5297-6740-7
ISBN 978-1-5297-6739-1 (pbk)

Contents

List of Figures and Tables

Figures

Tables

About the Editor and Contributors

The Editor

Annette Chowthi-Williams is an experienced academic, senior NHS manager and practitioner, and is currently an academic at the University of Roehampton in London. Dr. Chowthi-Williams is a Senior Fellow of the Higher Education Academy and an External Examiner. She has a particular interest in healthcare innovation and improvement, leadership, community and primary care and public health. Her interest in healthcare innovation and improvement has led to the development of possibly the first healthcare change management model in nursing and nurse education, and recently published a book on the subject, *Successful Change Management in Health Care: Being Emotionally and Cognitively Ready*. She is passionate about student wellbeing and on engaging and involving students in their teaching and learning.

The Contributors

Victoria Adebola is a Senior Lecturer and course leader at the University of West London. Her specialist areas encompass public health, acute medicine and surgery. Her clinical experience includes working in the United Kingdom and in Africa. She is working collaboratively with partner colleges linked with the university as part of the widening participation and academic partnerships engagement initiative. Her interest is in public health, particularly around maternal and child health and wellbeing. She has an MSc in International Child Health and is a Fellow of the Higher Education Authority. She is a champion for enhancing student experience and wellbeing and collaborates with academic and clinical colleagues to raise awareness of the importance of promoting student wellbeing in placement and in the university.

Daniela Blumlein is a Senior Lecturer in Adult nursing at the University of West London, and she has a passion for supporting students and helping them to maintain their wellbeing while studying. She is currently the course leader for a cohort of BNurs Adult students and has previously been the course leader for the PG Dip programme in Nursing. Daniela is an experienced RGN who has practiced in both Germany and the United Kingdom. She has an MA in Lifelong Learning Theories from the Institute of Education and a PG Dip in Professional Research Methods. Her background is in rehabilitation, Huntington's disease and brain injury nursing.

Janet Goddard is a Senior Lecturer and the Course Leader for Social Work at the University of West London. She completed the Transitioning to Leadership programme and is a Senior Convenor with the GMB. She specialises in teaching law, given her legal background and is also a trained Aromatherapist and Reflexologist. She is a Mentor and Coach and is a Lead Personal Tutor. Her interests are education and learning, mental health, dementia, assisted suicide and jurisprudence. Janet is a Fellow of the Higher Education Authority, a Fellow of the Royal Society for Public Health and a Member of the Chartered Institute of Arbitrators, specialising in mediation.

Regina Holley is a Senior Lecturer for Adult nursing and is currently the Course Leader for the Registered Nurse Degree Apprenticeship at the University of West London. She is a qualified nurse and midwife who has worked in Higher education for the last 20 years. She teaches across the pre-registration and post-registration courses.

Regina's experience in nursing and education spans 40 years and includes work overseas providing care services in a region of Nigeria with limited resources. She has also taught and supported adult literacy overseas and in the United Kingdom. Apart from her passion for education, Regina is a certified hypnotherapist who has a keen interest in personal wellbeing and resilience building.

Raquel Marta is currently a Senior Lecturer in Social Work at the University of West London. Dr. Marta has lectured widely on social work at undergraduate and postgraduate levels in the United States and Europe. Her social worker role involved focusing on the development and implementation of harm reduction policies and macro social work practice. Her research interests are creativity, complex thought, emotion and vulnerability with a particular focus on professional transformative abilities. Currently, her primary scholarly agenda are human development and environmental sustainability focusing on understanding individual vulnerabilities and their linkages with structural environmental inequalities in informal human settlements. Raquel is a member of the Children's Environments Research Group, the Center for Human Environments at the Graduate Center of the City University of New York and is affiliated with the International Federation of Social Work.

Ramona Minette Ramona Minette is a Senior Lecturer and Course Leader at the University of West London for students studying BNursing Adult Nursing. She is an experienced registered Adult and Mental Health Nurse. Experience includes acute surgery and orthopaedic nursing, medicine and acute mental healthcare for individuals with schizophrenia, self-harm and attempted suicide. Her research interests include Dementia, Stroke, Breast Cancer and Diabetes. She is currently the Lead for Recruitment and Selection of nursing and healthcare students with a keen interest in education, widening participation and promoting equality and diversity among students in the classroom and in practice. She is currently studying HEA Fellowship.

Kate Nash is an experienced clinician, Professional Midwifery Advocate (PMA) and academic, having held many varied roles and responsibilities within healthcare in London, the Midlands and the Southeast of England. Dr. Nash currently works as a Senior Lecturer at the University of the West of England and is passionate about enabling the development of the attitudes, skills and knowledge required for professional, safe and compassionate care provision. Kate has a keen interest in quality improvement and is committed to creating a supportive environment which provides opportunity for reflection and learning and where quality improvement initiatives can flourish.

Cathy Rowan is an experienced Senior Lecturer in midwifery on the 3-year pre-registration midwifery degree programme. She also co-leads the Examination of the Newborn post-registration module. She has a particular interest in perinatal mental health and leads a module on Holistic care for women and families with diverse psychosocial issues. Her research interest is around depression in immigrant women. She has previously published research in mental health provision and on problem-based learning in Midwifery.

Acknowledgements

I am extremely grateful to all my co-authors. It has been a real pleasure working with every one of you. Thank you for the hard work and dedication. It is no easy task meeting the deadline while at the same time dealing with the COVID-19 pandemic, working and undertaking family responsibilities.

A special thank you to my children, my granddaughter, husband, all my brothers, sisters, nieces, nephews and my son-in-law. A special thank you to my parents who, as always, are my inspiration.

Introduction

Annette Chowthi-Williams

What is This Book About and Who Should Read It?

This book was conceived after years of experience supporting health and social care students during their studies. With our combined experiences, we have gained invaluable knowledge and insights into the needs of health and social care students, and the importance of ensuring these needs are met. Most students entering university often find it challenging with the many adjustments they have to make. However, health and social care students programme of study have both theory and practice, thus not only do they have to adjust to university life but to the many practice settings both in hospitals and in community and primary care.

In the context of university, students are having to adapt to the language of university life and the healthcare world, new living environments, new forms of assessments, new ways of teaching and learning, emotional, physical and psychological challenges and towards becoming autonomous learners. The practice aspect of their course means that they are in a caring role, though under supervision. This means they have a level of responsibilities for the health and wellbeing of patients, service users and clients, sometimes with complex health needs as well as practicing in challenging settings. They also have the added responsibility of assessment of their practice. They usually will be working with and liaising with a range of teams and professional disciplines, and many students may be mature students with a family and some students may be studying a long way from their home.

These adjustments can be overwhelming for many students and poses a risk to their wellbeing. We have come to believe that supporting the wellbeing of students is paramount, if they are to provide safe, ethical and high-quality care for their patients, clients and service users. The wellbeing of students has not always been a priority in education or practice but there has been much learning from experience and evidence that students' wellbeing should be given the highest attention. The statutory bodies for the education and training of healthcare professional now recognise the need to consider students' wellbeing.

This book is an essential resource for health and social care students in nursing including midwives, social work and allied professionals starting a professional course. We have tried to write it in a student-friendly manner. It provides students with a host of general and specific resources to help, support, improve and maintain their wellbeing. It explores the many challenges students might encounter throughout their course of study and discusses the evidence on the impacts of these challenges and addresses how their holistic needs could be met. As the editor of this book, I hope you will find this book engaging, enjoyable and beneficial. I hope it will positively make a difference to your personal wellbeing now and in the future.

The Structure of This Book

This book consists of ten chapters. In each chapter, we have set out the aims, so that students know what is expected. There is an introduction to each chapter and a summary at the end of each chapter. In each chapter, there are learning features. We recognise that learning only from reading the literature can be perplexing especially when you have just started your course. Thus, to enable you to learn more effectively, we have set out activities, case studies scenarios, references, helpful links and resources that you can access easily to support your learning. This way of learning helps to develop independent learning and will help towards putting theory into practice. Naturally, no book can provide the answers to everything, but it is hoped that it will lead you towards the journey you wish to take in order to support, improve and maintain your wellbeing.

The activities will help to develop a range of skills. We ask you to reflect, to research information and to think critically. You will need to work with fellow students on some activities; this will help to develop your communication, teamwork, problem-solving, conflict resolution and reflective skills. You will be assessing your own needs, putting in place an action plan, implementing that plan and monitoring your progress. We hope the content of this book will help towards developing your planning, organisational, goal setting and evaluation skills as well as build your confidence, all of which are key skills needed for your profession.

Chapter 1

'The idea of being on a health and social care professional course was unnerving, but I would not change it for any other profession.'

In this first chapter, we would like to give you a flavour of university life in the context of health and social care studies. We will set out the unique nature of being a student on a professional course and consider some of the joys and challenges you might encounter as you grow and develop into a professional in your chosen field. This will include an overview of the academic team, your course, the importance of engaging yourself in your learning and academic integrity. We will consider the adjustments you may need to make that are innate to such courses and give you some ideas of how to develop yourself to meet these conditions. These adjustments might be emotional, financial, social, intellectual, cultural as well as the relationship between students and the professionals around you. We further consider life both as a young and mature student, leaving home, and managing family life. Finally, we will explore social media, online learning and becoming a part of the community of students and, subsequently, working professionals.

Chapter 2

'I found my 'calling' being on placement and I now know where I would like
to work when I finish the course.'

In this chapter, we delve into life in professional practice. Practice is the place where
you will be putting theory into action and is often referred to as 'placement'. We will
attempt to give you an overview of the practice aspect of your course in health and
social care and address the issues in a way that will be helpful to you. We will outline
what professional practice means, the actual and potential challenges and opportunities of caring for patients, clients and service users in a variety of settings where
you will be practicing your profession. We will consider ways of working and getting
the most out of your placement, being a learner, identifying your learning needs,
the essential role of supervision in practice and the importance of preparation for
practice. Being on placement can have a negative outcome and we explore this
aspect and reasons for disengagement of learners in practice. Finally, throughout
this chapter, we provide you with strategies, practical tips and solutions to aid your
life in professional practice as a health and social care student.

Chapter 3

In this chapter, we will explore the concept of wellbeing in general, in relation to
staying well as a student on a health and social care course, and outline the benefits of
wellbeing, in particular a high level of wellbeing. We will discuss factors that can
positively or negatively impact on a person's wellbeing and address how this may
apply to those in the caring professions. Healthcare workers often look after the
wellbeing of their clients, patients and service users but may not focus on their own
personal needs which may lead to them feeling stressed and less resilient. We will
explore the strategies, tools and resources to support personal wellbeing and will offer
some suggestions for self-care and maintaining or improving personal wellbeing for
health and social care students, as well as signposting sources for further support.

Chapter 4

Our mind, consciousness and emotions are linked, and it is important to understand
these connections. In this chapter, we will begin by exploring the nature of the
mind and how it is embodied in the interactions we have with others and the
environment. The discussion goes on to identify nurturing mind strategies to
cultivate wellbeing and it will help you to develop a robust understanding of
emotions and their impact on behaviour and responses to situations. In the final
part of the chapter, we will explore the workings of the mind and emotion and
consider strategies to optimise positive wellbeing and limit maladaptive emotional
responses, particularly in the social setting of the workplace. We will invite you to

reflect on your own emotional resources and to begin to consider strategies to strengthen them. We will have activities to engage with and scenarios to underpin your engagement with critical thinking, which is a skill that will serve you well on your professional course.

Chapter 5

We will begin in this chapter with exploring the nature of caring and what it means to you. We will consider the impact of the emotions that may be involved with caring and encourage you to reflect upon your emotional responses to help you understand your emotions and recognise how they might influence your own wellbeing. We will explore how your emotions might also influence your professional behaviour and the care you provide within practice. On an individual basis your emotional responses will be different depending on your background, circumstances, personality and previous experiences. We will consider various strategies that may be used to help you manage your emotions in a professional context. Various activities and case studies will be used to support the discussion throughout this chapter.

Chapter 6

In this chapter, we consider the question of what is emotional intelligence and explore some basics of emotional intelligence to help you understand the major characteristics and gain insight into how to nurture the development of emotional self-strategies. With leadership being a core skill for health and social care professional, how we come to incorporate skills and abilities derived from emotional intelligence into leadership in professional practice will also be discussed and explored. An essential foundation for a successful professional performance is the awareness of what emotions are; how they can be managed, developed and used in ourselves and in others. Emotions are part of our daily life and, as social and healthcare students and future leaders, it is essential that you nurture emotional intelligence both in your professional and personal life. We provide strategies and resources to help to become emotionally intelligent.

Chapter 7

This chapter will examine the notion of resilience, its role and importance in enabling students to manage and deal with challenges, drawbacks and the unexpected. It will explore the research within the field of resilience and offer a step-by-step guide to developing resilience. Building upon the concepts of emotional intelligence, this chapter will consider how practitioners can foster the skills for developing resilience as a strategy for managing challenges and enhancing emotional wellbeing within the workplace. The importance of building and maintaining resilience is stressed with available resources to support these aspects.

Chapter 8

In this chapter, we want to put the spotlight on your physical health. There is urgency to engage you in caring for yourselves and maintaining your physical health. Your physical health is linked to other aspects of your health and caring for your physical health will have a bearing on your mental, psychological and social health. The chapter will begin with defining health and exploring the potential challenges for health and social care students. We then give you an overview of the impact of physical activity on the anatomy and physiology of the body. Physical health is impacted by a range of sources such as healthy eating, good rest and sleep, a thriving social, community and family support, much relaxation and regular physical activities. We explore how to improve and maintain your physical health. We guide you through these elements and on how best to equip yourself with the right resources for the continued good physical health.

Chapter 9

In this chapter, we created some additional resources for you to enhance and maintain your wellbeing. We begin by reminding you that health needs to be viewed holistically and not to be separated into different components. We then continue the chapter with physical, mental and psychological and emotional health and the additional strategies and tools that you can access. There are three areas of health concern that we need to pay attention to in this chapter mainly because these are habits that can be challenging to manage and needs to be managed because of the impacts on our health and wellbeing. These are alcohol, smoking and obesity. We provide you with tools, resources and activities that you can access. Throughout this chapter, we refer to other chapters in this book where you can also find available resources so that you feel equipped to engage with your personal and professional growth and development.

Chapter 10

In this final chapter, we are keen to show you how to assess, implement, monitor and maintain your own personal wellbeing through creating your own journal. The first step in your personal wellbeing plan is to assess your current state of personal wellbeing and we have provided you with an assessment tool to do so. Once you have completed this, you will gain a picture of the level of your own personal wellbeing. Using this evidence of your present wellbeing, you can then take the next step of setting an action plan to improve your personal wellbeing. We have created an example to illustrate how you can go about setting your goals and steps to achieve your goals. While implementing your action, you could regularly monitor and review of your progress and if need be, re-set new goals. We will set out an array of resources available for you to access in order to improve and maintain your wellbeing while on your studies and beyond.

Requirements for Pre-Registration for Nurses, Social Worker and Allied Professions

NMC Standards of Proficiency for Registered Nurses (NMC, 2018)

1 Being an accountable professional
2 Promoting health and preventing ill health
3 Assessing needs and planning care
4 Providing and evaluating care
5 Leading and managing nursing care and working in teams
6 Improving safety and quality of care
7 Coordinating care

Professional Standards Social Work England (2019)

Standard 1: Promote the rights, strengths and wellbeing of people, families, and communities
Standard 2: Establish and maintain the trust and confidence of people
Standard 3: Be accountable for the quality of my practice and the decisions I make
Standard 4: Maintain my continuing professional development
Standard 5: Act safely and with professional integrity
Standard 6: Promote ethical practices and report concerns

Standards of Proficiency (HCPC, 2018)

1 Be able to practise safely and effectively within their scope of practice
2 Be able to practise within the legal and ethical boundaries of their profession
3 Be able to maintain fitness to practise
4 Be able to practise as an autonomous professional, exercising their own professional judgement
5 Be aware of the impact of culture, equality and diversity on practice
6 Be able to practise in a non-discriminatory manner
7 Understand the importance of and be able to maintain confidentiality
8 Be able to communicate effectively
9 Be able to work appropriately with others
10 Be able to maintain records appropriately
11 Be able to reflect on and review practice
12 Be able to assure the quality of their practice
13 Understand the key concepts of the knowledge base relevant to their profession
14 Be able to draw on appropriate knowledge and skills to inform practice
15 Understand the need to establish and maintain a safe practice environment

1

Becoming a Health and Social Care Student

Janet Goddard, Ramona Minette and Annette Chowthi-Williams

NMC Standards of Proficiency for Registered Nurses (NMC, 2019)
Professional Standards Social Work England (2019)
Standards of Proficiency (HCPC, 2018)

Nursing & Midwifery Council

This chapter will address the following platforms and proficiencies:

1 Being an accountable professional
2 Promoting health and preventing ill health
3 Assessing needs and planning care
4 Providing and evaluating care
5 Leading and managing nursing care and working in teams
6 Improving safety and quality of care
7 Coordinating care

Social Work England

This chapter will address the following standards:

Standard 1: Promote the rights, strengths and wellbeing of people, families and communities

Standard 2: Establish and maintain the trust and confidence of people

Standard 3: Be accountable for the quality of my practice and the decisions I make

Standard 4: Maintain my continuing professional development

Standard 5: Act safely and with professional integrity

Standard 6: Promote ethical practices and report concerns

Health and Care Professional Council

This chapter will address the following proficiencies:

1 Be able to practise safely and effectively within their scope of practice
2 Be able to practise within the legal and ethical boundaries of their profession
3 Be able to maintain fitness to practise
4 Be able to practise as an autonomous professional, exercising their own professional judgement
5 Be aware of the impact of culture, equality and diversity on practice
6 Be able to practise in a non-discriminatory manner
7 Understand the importance of and be able to maintain confidentiality
8 Be able to communicate effectively
9 Be able to work appropriately with others
10 Be able to maintain records appropriately
11 Be able to reflect on and review practice
12 Be able to assure the quality of their practice
13 Understand the key concepts of the knowledge base relevant to their profession
14 Be able to draw on appropriate knowledge and skills to inform practice
15 Understand the need to establish and maintain a safe practice environment

---

Chapter aims

After reading this chapter, you will be able to:

- Understand university life as a future health and social care professional.
- Demonstrate an awareness of what being a professional will mean for you.
- Describe what the requirements and adjustments you might need to make.
- Understand what the requirements are for social media usage and recognise the impact of incorrect use of social media might be on you and your profession.

Introduction

'**The idea of being on a health and social care professional course was unnerving, but I would not change it for any other profession'.** In this first chapter, we would like to give you a flavour of university life in the context of health and social care studies. We will set out the unique nature of being a student on a professional course and consider some of the joys and challenges you might encounter as you grow and develop into a professional in your chosen field. This will include an overview of the academic team, your course, the importance of engaging yourself in your learning and academic integrity. We will consider the adjustments you may need to make that are innate to such courses and give you some ideas of how to develop yourself to meet these conditions. These adjustments might be emotional, financial, social, intellectual, cultural as well as the relationship between students and the professionals around you. We further consider life both as a young and mature student, leaving home and managing family life. Finally, we will explore social media, online learning and becoming a part of the community of students and subsequently, working professionals.

Welcome to university life

━━━━━━━━ ACTIVITY **1.1** ━━━━━━━━

Research

List five things you already know about life at university and about the course you are studying.

Enrolling onto a professional course is the first step towards enjoying a rewarding career. You may have chosen to be a nurse, social worker, a paramedic or one of the many professions in health and social care. Whatever your individual professional choice, the one common theme in all health and social care professional is that you are caring for vulnerable people in a variety of settings. In Chapter 2, we will be discussing these settings in more detail. You may be caring for people through their lifespan, from pre-conception to end of life. You may be caring for women during pregnancy, babies, children, young people, adults, older people, those with mental health challenges, learning disability, the vulnerable, the very ill and people at the end of life. You will be caring for people in acute and specialist hospitals, in the homes of patients, clients and service users', in nursing and residential homes, children's home, rehabilitation centres, general practitioner (GP) practices and other settings. The first contact that the vast majority of people will have with the health service is in primary care, their GP.

Your course will include both theory and practice. 'Practice' is where you put into action the theory you have learnt in university. You will encounter joys and challenges, possibly both in equal measure. However, you will have a range of support and strategies to aid you through your programme of study. You will learn more about professional practice and the plethora of resources at your disposal within your chosen university and professional practice in later chapters.

You may have a mixture of feelings about how it will be, how you will cope, the sort of work you might do and what the challenges might be. It is understandable that you will have some nervousness about embarking on your chosen career path, but it is important to balance any concerns with the world of opportunity that will open up before you (Ghisoni & Murphy, 2019). Health and social care are dynamic fields of practice upon which an important dimension of the societal wellbeing is built. This means that while you are studying for your degree, you are also developing knowledge and transversal skills that will allow you to respond to the profession's future challenges and needs.

You will gain a wide range of skills, including those connected to employability, which you may not have anticipated as part of your learning journey. Throughout the course, you will deepen your knowledge and understanding of health and social care and develop an appreciation of the theoretical framework that will underpin your wider learning. You will balance your theoretical understanding with real-life case studies and practical work in your placement opportunities that will mould you into a knowledgeable, educated, and accomplished professional ready to engage with your profession on graduation; alternatively, you might want to engage with further learning and consider a postgraduate course before joining the world of work (Holloway et al., 2020). Healthcare professions offer some of the most rewarding, exciting and satisfying opportunities to you and you will develop diverse skills when working with some of the most vulnerable people in society.

You will be:

- a change-maker, a problem-solver, an innovator, a researcher, a leader, a manager, a team player, team leader, advocator, a facilitator and many more roles will come your way as you grow into your profession
- you will enjoy progression opportunities, and one of the first steps is identifying and understanding your motivation so that you can develop a plan for yourself. The diagram below includes some points for consideration, but you may also have areas you wish to include that are important to you.

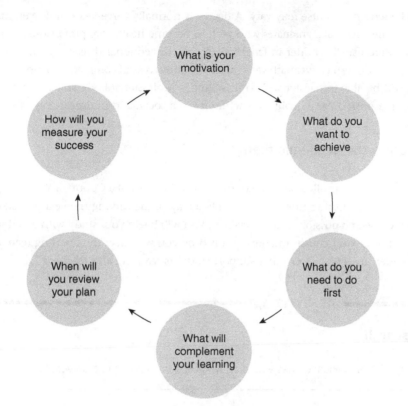

Figure 1.1 Self-reflection of your personal and professional needs

Your Course At University

Your health and social care course will have a specific length. You will be busy learning new skills, but you will also be expanding on your existing knowledge, changing and developing into a consummate professional (Nehrlich et al., 2019) and to enable that transition, your lessons will be theoretical and practical. The theoretical part of the course will be taught in your chosen university where you will be studying a range of subjects related to your profession from anatomy of the body, learning about diseases, what impacts people's health and wellbeing, how to improve people's health, caring for the sick and dying, to bringing about improvement and innovation in healthcare.

The practice element of your course will be in a variety of settings where you will be caring for people in the National Health Service (NHS), in the private sectors and in social care. You will not be expected to care for people on your own but will be under the wing of a more experienced professional in your field who will guide and support you. In the next chapter, you will learn more about your practice, often referred to as 'placement'.

The length of course may vary. A degree is normally three years; however, many universities now take graduates who wish to become healthcare professionals. These courses are usually shorter in length than the conventional three years degree and more intense. Whichever pathway you chose, on successful completion of your study, you will be able to register with your statutory professional body and you can then take up a position as a qualified practitioner in a social and healthcare organisation.

Meeting the academic team

Once you have enrolled on your course, you will be part of a Cohort, a Year group or there may be another title. This is simply a way of identifying the year you started your course and possibly your specialism. You will begin your study with a period of induction to your course and during this time you will meet the teaching team and the wider university teams that support students learning and teaching.

━━━━━━━━━━ ACTIVITY 1.2 ━━━━━━━━━━

Research

Make a list of academic titles you already know that teaches in a university.

You will be given a personal tutor (PT) who will support you during your study and you will meet your personal tutor at regular intervals, but you can contact your personal tutor anytime you need to. You will meet a range of people supporting your study, module leaders, programme leaders, course directors, lecturers, senior lecturers, doctors, professors, placement or practice teams, programme administrators and the wider university teams that provide student support such as the library, ICT, student wellbeing, academic development, finance, student union and the host of other teams supporting students. You will be given more details about the course, the subjects, topics or modules you will be studying each year and the various resources at the university that you can access anytime.

You will be given online access to your course, the learning materials and resources. You will receive a plan of your three years of study showing dates when theory will begin and end, together with placement dates but not actual placement name. Your three years plan will also have dates of holiday leave and study time. You will see your timetable which will be packed with lessons, independent, and guided independent work, all of which will need to be factored into your week. You will need to become very organised and plan your week well, so that you do not fall behind with your work which will be unnecessarily stressful (Hallam et al., 2018).

You will see that you will have to complete assessments for each module on your course. You will be assessed in a variety of innovative ways (Carless, 2015); for example, you might have traditional exams and coursework, but you will also undertake role play, presentations, group work, reflections, portfolios, listen to podcasts and oral assessments (Cottrell, 2019). This allows your chosen university to assess you in diverse ways so that everyone has an equal opportunity to excel.

You will have set dates to complete your essays, and these will be published well in advance to give you time to plan your assessments. It is essential that you submit these on time as delays mean you may not be able to move to the next year or qualify on time. However, there may be circumstances beyond your control which means that you may not be able to submit your essay on the set dates. In such situations, you should contact your module leader immediately and inform them of your situation. All universities will allow you to apply for an extension or mitigation, if you have a reason as to why you cannot submit your assignment on time. What is absolutely essential is that you communicate with all key people on your course, if you cannot complete your work on the required date and time.

Engagement and involvement In your learning

It is essential when you begin your course, you engage in and with your learning. It is also essential that the university you are studying with make every effort to engage you as a student. Many experts have written and researched the subject of student engagement.

There is evidence that student engagement has positive outcomes for student and disengagement can lead to negative outcomes. However, you may well be asking the question what is student engagement? What does this mean for me undertaking a health and social care course? Experts have sought to define the idea of student engagement. Skinner and Belmont (1993, p. 572) defined student engagement as 'sustained behavioural involvement in learning activities accompanied by positive emotional tone'. Another team of experts believe that 'Student engagement is the energy and effort that students employ within their learning community. The more students are engaged and empowered within their learning community, the more likely they are to channel that energy back into their learning, leading to a range of short- and long-term outcomes, that can likewise further fuel engagement' (Bond et al., 2020, p. 3). These experts believe that those students who are involved and engaged in their learning attain better achievement and are more purposeful towards their studies, and such students are more likely to stay on the course. Whereas students who do not involve themselves in their learning could experience negative effects to their learning, their cognitive development and may lose interest in their studies.

Engagement in your learning begins as soon as you embark on your course, as you progress through it and as you are approaching the end. Engagement in your teaching and learning, assessment and your course curriculum are a joint responsibility between you and your university. You should make active efforts to be proactive in your learning.

Your university should engage you through ensuring that students on your course are represented on their various boards and committees. They also need to actively share their ideas on how they want you to engage with them (Bryson, 2014; Buckley, 2014). Some universities may set out agreements on engagement, provide you with resources on how you can become engaged with your place of study, others might facilitate workshops, conversations, events, activities and forums. Try to get to one or all of these activities to learn about how to get engaged in your studies.

Case study 1.1

James

After failing his coursework on the second attempts, James was in shock, citing that he doesn't understand why he has failed, after all he has been reading all the teaching material and he read the assignment guidance carefully. No need to be at lectures was James's view.

============== **ACTIVITY 1.3** ==============

Research

What do you think, should students attend lectures?

Why might attendance to lectures benefit you?

Are there reasons for not attending lectures?

It is important to be aware that learning is more than reading the learning material. Attendance to lecture regularly is a key part of learning and this would have helped James to understand the learning material better through joining in the classroom activities, discussions and presentations. He might have picked up ideas from the group or from individuals about the assignment or on ways of studying. Being present in lectures would have allowed him to ask pertinent questions, clarify anything he didn't understand, have a one-to-one discussion with the lecturer on his assignment plan, then shared his draft plan and get feedback, all of which could have aided his motivation. Through engaging in his learning, he would have also received advice on academic support or other kinds of support if he had concerns and worries.

Tips for engaging in your learning:

- In lessons, join in group discussions, activities and presentations.
- Research your subject and if you feel you are not grasping your subject matter, discuss your thoughts with the module or subject leader.
- Ask questions and don't apologise for asking, it is what learning is all about. If you knew the subject matter, you would not be embarking on the course.
- Be a course representative on the university course committees

- Be active in the student union
- Join a community of learning group on your course
- Set up your own study group
- Find out what support your university is offering on engaging student and seek such support
- Join in physical, cultural and other activities

Academic integrity

We outlined earlier that during the duration of your course, you will have theoretical and practice exams to undertake for each of your modules. You will be given dates well in advance when various coursework, exams and practical exams will take place. You may be required to engage in a viva to verbally discuss your work, or you may have to attend an Academic Offences Panel, where more serious penalties may be attached to the outcome if it is upheld. If it is very serious or a repeated offence, your place in the course may be placed in jeopardy.

Thus, academic integrity is an essential requirement in academia, and every university will have academic regulations you should read. Academic integrity refers to complete honesty in your work, which means you should acknowledge the work of others, by giving them credit. There are processes in place to address breaches of academic regulations as it brings into question your personal integrity. It is considered as cheating to gain advantage and will be addressed accordingly. In order to safeguard yourself from this risk, you need to understand what constitutes academic misconduct. Do you think you know what constitutes academic misconduct?

Below are a few scenarios for you to read. Think about whether you believe they would be considered as academic misconduct or not.

━━━━━━━━ **SCENARIO** 1.1 ━━━━━━━━

You get consent in writing from Bob to use his work in your paper. You use his work as you have his consent and do not cite him as you have an agreement in place with him. **Yes/No**

You write your paper, and you cite all of your sources using the wrong referencing system (see link below). For example, you use APA when it should be Harvard. **Yes/No**

You are asked to write a similar paper to one you wrote in college. You received a good grade and decide to update the paper and submit it for the assignment. You are not concerned as it is all your own work. **Yes/No**

You are working late into the evening on your paper and have found most of the references and cited them correctly. There are two diagrams in your paper you cannot find the reference for, so you just refer to a book you have used more generally throughout your work. **Yes/No**

You work with one of your peers on a paper that you are both finding difficult. You both work hard and make certain the papers are not too similar. **Yes/No**

Answers at the end of this chapter.

Making adjustments into university life

The transition from your present situation into university life will mean inevitable adjustments in a number of ways. Not only for you but your family and friends. Entering university is a change and any change, be it personal or professional to our life, will mean making adjustments. Leaving home and parting from family, friends and everything that has been familiar to you to move to university can feel challenging and, possibly, overwhelming.

Case study 1.2

Fredo

Fredo was the eldest child in the family and grew up with a very supportive family. He was very close to his brother and two sisters. He and his family were absolutely delighted on receiving the news that he can begin the course to become a paramedic. He was the first in the family to go to university. But as the time became closer for him to leave home and begin his studies, he found himself feeling anxious and questioning whether he had made the right decision to study so far from home.

ACTIVITY 1.4

Reflection and Research

Can you think of reasons why Fredo might be feeling anxious?

Write down your reasons and discuss these with your peers.

When you begin university life, it is inevitable that there will be many changes to your life and circumstances. You may not have thought about such matters previously. However, you may find that there are many adjustments you may need to make such as academic, cultural, emotional, financial, intellectual and social (Hazard & Carter, 2018).

Academic adjustment may mean a change in the way you have been learning. You will have been used to your own ways of study. Your course will involve the need to understanding unfamiliar materials, activities and complex information. Entering university will entail new ways of learning, more independent learning, using technology and other resources. Seeking help early is important. Most universities will have resources such as academic support with writing at the right level and libraries will have a range of resources to support your learning.

Cultural change is part of university life. These institutions have their own language and customs, and thus you may need to learn these and what they mean in the context of your study may. For example, modules, programmes, lectures, tutorials and simulation. Get ahead and read up in advance. You will meet people from diverse backgrounds, encounter new kinds of cuisine, cultural activities. Join in and experience these wonderful new activities.

Emotional adjustment can be challenging and could be one of the most difficult changes you may encounter. You are bound to feel stressed, worried and at times may question your choice. You will miss your family, friends and your familiar surroundings. These are all normal feelings. Join in the activities such a gym, yoga or if you prefer an online activity to help reduce stress. Talk to a counsellor or ask for help at the student support desk. Talk with friends on the course, your personal tutor and the student union.

Intellectually, you will be learning many new theories, discover new and exciting ideas which will stimulate your thinking and your feelings. Your thinking and feelings will be challenged. You may need to adjust to the different levels of course. As you move up and towards your final year, your course might feel tougher and to be expected. You will be studying at a higher level and expected to be much more analytical, read more widely and use a wider body of evidence to support your work. Seek help from the many sources we have already suggested.

Social adjustment can be exciting and daunting at the same time. You will be meeting new people in university and in practice. You will encounter new settings and yet more new people, teams and different disciplines. You will build new relationships and at times these will be challenging. You will need to learn how to successfully manage these and use the university support network that will be in place.

Financial worries may be inevitable or not and this will depend on your specific and personal circumstances. It is essential to know what is available and how to apply for support. To help prevent delays, have all your documents to hand and take time to complete any necessary forms. The cost of living in studying in the United Kingdom is one of the most crucial factors for international students to give special attention to this issue, and for all students to bear in mind that any capital city will be more costly.

Will my peer group all be older or younger than me?

Sometimes we forget that education, growth and development is not the preserve of any one group but, rather, it is a collective aspiration, and we gain a wider understanding when we mix with others outside of our normal family, friends and age groups.

One of the approaches universities promote is lifelong learning, and it is also part of the professional bodies' requirements and advancement of the field (Craig et al., 2019; Ramscar et al., 2014) because we know that we benefit from a good education as we have the potential to find different or better jobs, become more successful in our career and expand our prospects. It is important to recognise, however, that formal education is only one element of learning, another being our experiences which we can share, grow and develop from. We can think of it as engaging and growing by imaginative or sympathetic participation in the experiences of others.

There is no age requirement or limit to this as we all learn from each other when we recognise that learning does not flow in one direction only. It is important to acknowledge the rapid and continuous changes that occur in the medical and social fields, which may be regulatory, legal and political (Gov.uk, 2017), so what we need to do then is develop our curiosity, our skills and a positive attitude to learning for personal and professional development, but also, for the simple enjoyment of investing in ourselves.

———————— ACTIVITY 1.5 ————————

Reflection and Critical Thinking

Think about your own reasons for learning. What are you hoping to achieve?

For example:

Do you want to:

- Increase your learning and skillset?
- Advance in your career?
- Change your career?
- Develop new skills?
- Become more self-sufficient?
- Do you just want to experience the joy of learning?

Now create a plan considering the following: (remember this can change, so do not feel you are setting inflexible or unchangeable goals that will bind you)

- What are the first steps you need to take?
- Do you have a short-term, mid-term and long-term plan?
- Think about complementary skills because employers want to see transferable skills too; so, make sure you factor these into your plan.
- Finally, think of the things that are motivating you to succeed because when you feel as if you are struggling, your motivation will help you to refocus and re-engage.

Social media

It is forecast that social media users will reach almost 51 million by 2025, which accounts for a market penetration of around 73.5%, so you can see that many of us are engaged in using social media in some form. While it is important to recognise the positive aspects of using social media, as it can transform the way services are delivered, we must also acknowledge we need to develop a robust understanding of data protection before posting on any site, to prevent harm to others (Reamer, 2013; Shi et al., 2019). We are generally aware of what social media are and we may have a personal relationship with it on some level, but we need to think about it slightly differently when it comes to becoming a professional as it can have a significant effect if we use it incorrectly (McGrath et al., 2019; The British Association of Social Workers, 2018). Your engagement and commitment with a health and/or social care course implies a full commitment with ethical professional values and standards and so understanding the risk is invaluable before engaging on any social media platform. The use of social media sites with your student peer group is equally not without risk, because once you post something, you lose control of it which might be damaging to yourself and/or others; for example, someone may be offended by something you say, take a screenshot of it, and use it in a complaint, which might impact your position on the course (Ramage and Moorley, 2019). So, while social media can be useful for sharing information immediately with each other, it can also be harmful as it can be where people create an endless stream of stress, give incorrect information or discuss matters that might potentially breach data protection. Engage with the activities below and consider what the issues might be. You can check your response afterwards to see if you were correct.

Case study 1.3

John

John has created a group WhatsApp page for his colleagues so that they can share information about an upcoming presentation. John has arranged to see the tutor on Wednesday about a personal matter and, afterwards, his entire group is meeting the tutor to discuss their work. On Tuesday, the tutor informs John through email that she is unwell and will not be able to see him. She asks John to inform his group that she will be unable to meet them but will reset the meeting as soon as possible. John decides to share the email on WhatsApp. When the tutor returns and finds that John has shared the email, she is very angry and asks to see him to ask why he decided to do it without her permission. John thought he could share the email as she had asked him to inform the group.

ACTIVITY 1.6

Critical Thinking

- Was John right or wrong to share the email?
- What should John have done first?
- What do you think the right outcome should have been?
- Why?

Case study 1.4

Rosemary

Rosemary is a member of John's group and was preparing the presentation with the rest of the group. She realised that she has everyone's mobile number, except for Stephen's, so she is unable to check whether he has finished his slides. Ben has Stephen's number and posts it on the group with everyone else's number so that they can all contact each other. When Stephen finds out Ben has shared his number in the WhatsApp group, he raises a complaint with the Course Leader. Stephen deliberately chose to not share his number as he knew they could contact him via email. The Course Leader addresses the matter with Ben as he has shared Stephen's number without consent. Do you think the outcome was right or wrong?

Case study 1.5

Outcome

John was in the wrong. While he had authority to share the tutor was not coming in, he did not have permission to share that she was unwell. Before sharing the email, John should have asked for permission to share, or he should have simply informed the group she was not able to meet with them and would reset the meeting. Before sharing information, check that you have permission or consent to share. If you do not, you could find yourself in a difficult position, which could be addressed legally, if it was serious enough, so always check first.

Case study 1.6

Outcome

Ben should not have shared Stephen's personal information without consent regardless of the fact that they were in the same group. The information could have been shared by Stephen if he had wanted everyone to have it. Ben should have sought permission before making the decision to share Stephen's private details, rather than deciding to share it without consent. The university was right to respond to the breach.

Finally, please make sure you also do your own research for any other information you need, as there are several sites that may help you.

Chapter Summary

In this introductory chapter, we are keen to give you a taste of university life and the future opportunities as you begin your chosen course of study. We have tried to give you an overview of the specifics of health and social care courses. Such courses involve caring for people in different settings and contain theory and practice, both of which are assessed through a variety of means such as exams, coursework, simulation, observation, presentations and practical exams. We have introduced you to some of the language of university life as you meet the academic team and stressed the importance of engaging in your learning and ensuring that you maintain academic integrity. Naturally, there will be change as you leave all that is familiar to you and enter university. We have set out the potential adjustments you may need to make and offer some tips to help you adjust to the change. There may be concerns about your peer group, but it is important that you focus on your reasons for wanting to become a health and social care profession. We ended the chapter with a discussion around social media which can pose particular hazards to yourself and your chosen profession. It is essential that you pay attention to this growing area of concern and always act professionally in line with the code of practice of your professional body.

Answer to Academic Integrity

No	Yes	No
1	Even though you have his agreement in place, you still need to cite him as it is his work, rather than your own. This would be considered as plagiarism, which is taking someone's work and passing it off as your own.	
2		It is not likely to be considered as academic misconduct, but it is poor academic practice as you should have made certain of the referencing system your course uses. In future, you would need to follow the referencing guidelines for your course.
3	This is academic misconduct. Although it is your own work, it was previously submitted and graded and would be considered as self-plagiarism, or, cheating to gain advantage.	
4	This is academic misconduct, as it is a false citation.	
5	This is academic misconduct, as you are colluding on a paper without agreement. Any work submitted must be entirely your own.	

2

Life in Professional Practice

Annette Chowthi-Williams
and Janet Goddard

NMC Standards of Proficiency for Registered Nurses (NMC, 2018)
Professional Standards Social Work England (2019)
Standards of Proficiency (HCPC, 2018)

Nursing & Midwifery Council

This chapter will address the following platforms and proficiencies:

1 Being an accountable professional
2 Promoting health and preventing ill health
3 Assessing needs and planning care
4 Providing and evaluating care
5 Leading and managing nursing care and working in teams
6 Improving safety and quality of care
7 Coordinating care

Social Work England

This chapter will address the following standards:

Standard 1: Promote the rights, strengths and wellbeing of people, families and
communities
Standard 2: Establish and maintain the trust and confidence of people
Standard 3: Be accountable for the quality of my practice and the decisions I make
Standard 4: Maintain my continuing professional development
Standard 5: Act safely and with professional integrity
Standard 6: Promote ethical practices and report concerns

Health and Care Professional Council

This chapter will address the following proficiencies:

1 Be able to practise safely and effectively within their scope of practice
2 Be able to practise within the legal and ethical boundaries of their profession
3 Be able to maintain fitness to practise
4 Be able to practise as an autonomous professional, exercising their own professional
   judgement
5 Be aware of the impact of culture, equality and diversity on practice
6 Be able to practise in a non-discriminatory manner
7 Understand the importance of and be able to maintain confidentiality
8 Be able to communicate effectively
9 Be able to work appropriately with others
10 Be able to maintain records appropriately
11 Be able to reflect on and review practice
12 Be able to assure the quality of their practice
13 Understand the key concepts of the knowledge base relevant to their profession
14 Be able to draw on appropriate knowledge and skills to inform practice
15 Understand the need to establish and maintain a safe practice environment

---

Chapter aims

After reading this chapter, you will be able to:

- Gain knowledge and understanding of the role and importance of clinical placement as
  a trainee.
- Understand the role of your supervisor and academic assessor/education team.
- Understand the challenges of being a learner in the clinical setting.
- Understand how to manage teamwork/conflicts/challenging situations.
- Gain knowledge on coping strategies for dealing with clinical/practice challenges.

Introduction

I found my 'calling' being on placement and I now know where I would like to work when I finish the course. In this chapter, we delve into life in professional practice. Practice is the place where you will be putting theory into action and is often referred to as 'placement'. We will attempt to give you an overview of the practice aspect of your course in health and social care and address the issues in a way that will be helpful to you. We will outline what professional practice means, the actual and potential challenges and opportunities of caring for patients, clients and service users and the variety of settings where you will be practising your profession. We will consider ways of working and getting the most out of your placement, being a learner, identifying your learning needs, the essential role of supervision in practice and the importance of preparation for practice. Being on placement can have a negative outcome and we explore this aspect and reasons for disengagement of learners in practice. Finally, throughout this chapter, we provide you with strategies, practical tips and solutions to aid your life in professional practice as a health and social care student.

What is Professional Practice

Health and social care students undertake practice alongside the theory part of their course. In effect, practice is where theory is put into action. The practice element of the course is usually referred to as **'student placement'**, 'practice placement' or simply 'placement'. Placement is where you will be practising your craft and doing so in a variety of settings. Starting professional practice can and will seem overwhelming to new students but your universities will ensure that they prepare you for placements which should help to ease any anxieties.

Your 'placement' will be in a variety of settings that provides care for patients, clients and service users. You are expected to abide by your professional code of conducts, professional values, ethics and standards and maintain a professional relationship with your patients, clients and service users. You are thus accountable for your practice and should not undertake any aspect of care till you have been assessed as competent by the team supervising and assessing your practice. You will be in an environment that you have possibly never experienced previously which will stimulate and excite you but also may pose challenges, stresses and anxieties you have not experienced before.

━━━━━━━━ ACTIVITY **2.1** ━━━━━━━━

Research and Reflection

Think about what would stimulate and excite you in placement.

Write these down.

Now think about what might pose a challenge for you and write these down.

You can expect to:

- work with an array of diverse professionals
- support, care for sick and dying patients in hospitals, in people's homes, clinics, schools, residential homes and GP practices
- understand and work with organisational structures and processes
- at times feel incompetent when undertaking procedures
- working with new and different teams across all disciplines
- achieve statutory professional values, practices and proficiencies set by your professional body
- negotiate yourself in what can seem like an alien environment.
- feel at times that there is a mismatch between theory and practice
- witness tough living conditions and lifestyles of your patients/service users and clients
- at times feel overwhelmed by the challenges some people may be facing with disability and illness

You will encounter many different kinds of health, social, economic, environmental, emotional, mental health and other conditions in practice. You will be caring for people:

- with challenging lives, in poor housing conditions, some people may be living in poverty
- exposed to violence on children and adults or at risks of abuse
- people with complex health needs and challenging patients
- who are lonely, especially older people and many others with a range of social and emotional needs
- who are at the end of life and death of people of all age range
- those recovering from operations, experiencing emergencies and trauma
- babies who are very ill and some with long-term illness
- people with disability, both adults and children

You will also experience:

- professional satisfaction, joy and happiness when patients recovered from illnesses and are discharged to their homes

- at the birth of a newborn, children progressing and developing healthily
- people recovering from emotional, mental health and psychological challenges
- people's successful recovery post-surgery and adapting to personal changes
- people successfully managing their health and wellbeing sometimes with disabling conditions
- at the end of successful placement, working with a proactive and supportive teams and other disciplines
- the share volume of support available in health and social care for patients, service users, clients and the workforce
- at the ingenuity, energy and innovation of both the people you care for and the carers

Where Does Practice Take Place?

You will have placements in a variety of settings. In these settings you will be preventing ill health and promoting good health and caring for people with a variety of health needs.

Community health services provide an extensive and diverse range of activities and support services across a range of needs and age groups. This service is used on a regular basis by children, older people, those living with frailty or chronic conditions and people who are near the end of their life. Community services support people with multiple and complex health needs. These patients, service users and clients generally are dependent on health and social care services to help meet their needs.

In this setting, professionals work in partnership with a range of other services within the National Health Service (NHS). These might be GPs, acute and specialist hospitals, community pharmacies and with nursing or residential homes. A major part of community services involves preventative services and may also include services such as prison and dentistry (Kings Fund, 2019). With many diseases now linked to lifestyle factors, preventing ill health and promoting good health is a critical part of the role of health and social care professionals in every setting. Your course will provide you with the knowledge and skills to help patients, service users and clients improve their health and wellbeing and prevent ill health.

Primary healthcare is the first point of contact for healthcare for the majority of the population. It is primarily provided by GPs and delivered in small, medium size and large GP practices. Usually, practices cover a particular population size for each GP. GP practices are spread across the country, and everyone should have a GP. There are services such as community pharmacists, opticians and dentists which are also primary healthcare providers (NHS England, 2022)

Local authorities have a major public health role. The Health and Social Care Act (2012) transferred public health from the NHS to local government. You will learn or may already know that there is an array of factors that impact the health and wellbeing of the population. These determinants of health include housing, unemployment, education, the work environment, healthcare services, socio-economic status and other factors (Danlgren & Whitehead, 1993). The change in healthcare policy puts councils across the country in a prime position to tackle these wider determinants of health through working with a variety of statutory, voluntary and private organisations. These include the NHS, charities, local community groups, community health services, other public-sector and independent organisations, and the population they are responsible for. A key role for councils is to engage and involve the population in the planning and delivering of services to improve the population's health. Services such as child health and sexual health which were once under the guise of the NHS have now been moved to local authorities. These include the health visiting (Specialist Community Public Health Nursing [SCPHN]) and school nursing services.

Private sector in the community and primary care setting generally involves the services provided by some nursing and residential homes for the population. These include services for children, young people to the elderly.

Thus within the context of community and primary care, you will be caring for people in these different organisations, services and settings. This includes caring for people in their homes, in rehabilitation centres, in nursing homes, children's homes, in GP practices, health centres, outreach clinics, mental health and learning disability homes and in specialist units. You will also be exploring the work of the voluntary sectors, charities and specialist organisations that care for the homeless, domestic violence, child protection, and many other organisations that provide care and support for older people, children, people with learning disability, mental health needs, women, men, young people and different ethnic and cultural groups.

Some of the current services in community and primary care and local authority

Targeted/specialist services

Range of community services

Child health
Community occupational therapy
Community paediatric clinic
Community palliative care
Community physiotherapy
Community podiatry
Community speech and language therapy
Dietician

District nursing
Falls service
Intermediate services
Specialist nursing services, i.e. diabetes, tissue viability, heart failure, incontinence
Wheelchair services

Universal public health function

Health visiting (SCPHN)
School nursing
Sexual health services

Possible placement settings

Rehabilitation centres
Patients' homes
Nursing homes — private sector and NHS
Charities, cultural and voluntary groups
Schools/playgroups/nurseries
Children's homes
GP practices
Health centres
Outreach clinics
Mental health and learning disability units

Acute sector: Hospitals across the country provide care and treatment for the population with a range of services. There are numerous hospitals both in the NHS and the private sector. Hospital care usually involve diagnosing illness, providing treatment and care and discharging patients, service users and clients back to their homes. In many instances, they continue monitoring people's health till full recovery or in some situations providing continuous treatment, for example, people receiving cancer treatment or people with long-term and complex conditions. The care and treatment provided is not just physical but mental, emotional and psychological, and hospitals often have a wide range of general and specialist services.

Specialised services support people with a range of rare and complex conditions. For example, according to NHS England, these treatments can be provided to patients with rare cancers, genetic disorders or complex medical or surgical conditions. Many have world leading research facilities and have an international reputation for innovative treatment and care in the NHS. They tend to be trailblazers and not only provide a range of treatments known to the public such as chemotherapy, radiotherapy and kidney dialysis but undertake groundbreaking interventions with a small number of patients. NHS England has given these examples, using a patient's own tooth to restore their sight and hand transplants. They are also involved in trials of treatment. You can learn more through the link below.

https://www.england.nhs.uk/commissioning/spec-services/

In a hospital setting, you would be placed in a number of different areas. Depending on your field, you could be placed in a children's, mental health or adult ward. These could be medical, surgical, elderly wards, in the accident and emergency, outpatient department (OPD), midwifery and specialist units.

Some of the many hospital services

General surgery
  General medicine
  Emergency care
  Out-patient
  Mental health services
  Children services
  Maternity services
  Learning disability
  Physiotherapy
  Occupational therapy
  Dietician
  Radiology
  Social work

Specialised services

Chemotherapy
  Radiotherapy
  Kidney dialysis
  Genetic conditions
  Transplants
  Watch the video below for the range of specialised services
  https://www.england.nhs.uk/commissioning/spec-services/

ACTIVITY 2.2

Research and Reflection

Think about the services in community and primary care and hospital setting.

Which setting do you think the majority of the population are cared for?

Have you any preference for a particular setting, if so, why?

Readiness for Practice: University Preparation

You will be given preparation for practice in a number of ways by your university before you start your practice placement. You will practice your skills in the university through 'simulation'. This means you will first be taught the theoretical aspects of care. For example, giving basic life support (BLS). This procedure will then be demonstrated by a lecturer (not on patients, service users or clients but on manikin designed for this purpose) after which you will then be given plenty of opportunity to practice. You will practice until you think and feel confident and competent. After which you will be assessed to ensure you are competent.

Your skills will also be assessed throughout your course through objective structured clinical examination (OSCE) to ensure you are continuing to be a safe practitioner on 'placement'. These assessments are usually undertaken by lecturers and usually planned well in advance. Again, there will be preparation sessions and you will know the criteria that are being used for your assessment.

Case study 2.1

Nana

During a simulation session on BLS, Nana suddenly became anxious about going into practice. She blurts out her thoughts to the groups. She expressed the view that she doesn't think she will ever be able to carry out such a procedure. She told the group she does not feel confident about her knowledge and skills even though she has had the opportunity to practice. She went on to say that she will never remember the procedure and will be sure to panic and get things wrong in 'placement'.

ACTIVITY 2.3

Reflection

How can you help Nana ease her worries?

What might you suggest to Nana to help ease her worries?

It is perfectly normal to feel anxious about readiness for your practice. However, these taught activities together with practice under supervision of lecturers and then assessment should build your confidence and competence to ensure readiness for practice. However, some of you may well feel daunted by the idea of clinical assessment in the university. Be assured, you will not be assessed on anything you have not been taught and you will get plenty of opportunities to practise before being assessed.

- Universities have a team to support you in practice. You will be given a named education or academic assessor from the university, who will support you in practice and work closely with your placement practice assessor and supervisor. We will tell you more about your practice supervisor and assessor later in this chapter. You will have a preparation on how you will be assessed in practice, the relevant documentation and the importance of recording and verifying your practice hours. Your professional proficiencies, values and practice that you need to achieve in placement will be set out in a document. In some professions, this is referred to as **Practice Assessment Document** (PAD). Many universities now have these electronically as **epad.** Your university team will spend time with you and the practice team to ensure everyone knows the significance of your epad or PAD and how to record your practice hours and the achievement of your proficiencies.

You will be given details of your practice placement and other details well in advance. This includes details on:

- your placement location and name of hospital/community and primary location and ward/clinic
- names of the practice team and contact details
- a start and end of your placement
- name and contact details of the education/academic assessor
- documentation (referred to as PAD or epad) with the relevant proficiencies to be achieved on placement.

On Placement: Supervision

We already informed you that your course consists of theory and practice and that the practice element of course will take place in different settings. We gave you details on these settings earlier in this chapter. We also stated that practice is often referred to as 'placement'. The length of time you spend in placement will depend on your profession. Later in the chapter, we have set out some information on the practice hours for different professional groups. The length of your placement will depend on your overall practice hours of your course and will be spread out over the lifetime of your course.

While you are on 'placement', you will be caring for patients, clients and service users under the supervision of an experienced practitioner, who will have years of experience and would have received extra education and training to support learners in practice. Different profession groups have different names for practitioners facilitating student learning in practice. Some professionals refer to these practitioners as practice supervisors, practice assessors, practice team or practice facilitators. Some professions, for example, nursing students have a practice supervisor, who supports students on a day-to-day basis and a practice assessor who will assess their professional proficiencies, values and practice and sign these off on the epad or PAD.

Once you begin placement, you will:

- be allocated a specific practitioner/practice supervisor/assessor to support your learning in practice and you will be given a full induction to your placement.
- not be expected to care for patients, clients and service users without the support and supervision of a qualified practitioner.
- first observe the experienced practitioners/supervisor caring for patients, service users and clients
- then undertake care under close supervision by your allocated practitioner/ supervisor/assessor in practice
- continue in your caring role under supervision till you and your supervisor think and feel you are fully competent
- then you will be assessed on the professional proficiencies, values and other aspects of care to ensure you are fully competent
- then these professional proficiencies, values and aspects of care will be signed off in your PAD or epad by your allocated practice assessor
- throughout your placement you will also meet with your academic assessor

In the acute sector, your practice supervisor and assessor may be:

- a qualified nurse or midwife
- a physiotherapist
- a dietician
- a speech and language therapist
- an occupational therapist
- a podiatrist
- a social worker
- a paramedic or
- a radiographer.

In community and primary care, this may be:

- a district nurse
- a health visitor
- a primary care nurse
- a specialist nurse
- a specialist mental health nurse
- a specialist practitioner or matron
- a practice nurse
- a community midwife
- a physiotherapist

- a dietician
- a speech and language therapist
- an occupational therapist
- a podiatrist
- a social worker or
- a radiographer.

In general, each student will have a team of practice staff and academics helping to support their learning in practice. This is beneficial to your learning as it means you have many sources of support.

Getting the Most Out of Supervisors and How to Be Proactive With Your Learning

The relationship with your supervisor/assessor is a crucial one, so try to work towards developing an effective working relationship. Remember supervisors/assessors are busy practitioners whose overriding priority will be the care of their patients, service users and clients. They are supervising you because they have years of experience and so to get the best from your placement, it is essential that you engage in your learning.

Here are some helpful tips:

- try to meet with the practice team before you start your placement
- undertake research about your hospital and ward, your neighbourhood, its population, their health needs a resources and support for service users, patients and clients
- have all your documentation to hand and discuss your learning needs with the practice team right at the start of your placement
- keeping the practice team informed if you going to be late, sick or experiencing any other challenges.
- be proactive and organise to meet the team on a regular basis, so that everyone can gauge your progress and offer opportunities to develop further
- reflect regularly on your learning and set yourself new goals with your allocated supervisor/assessor

Cultivating a Good Working Relationship With Peers and Other Professionals in Placement

Placement is a crucial part of your university path, allowing you to directly engage with practice learning in real-life settings while stimulating your further development, creating and managing new interpersonal relationships, increasing your level of responsibility and accountably and, naturally, creating additional challenges. Among the challenges associated is the importance of relationships.

Your relationship with those around you in placement is often dependent on your own engagement and investment in the tasks attributable to your chosen role and with the professionals there to support and work alongside you. It also includes, students from your own university and students from different institutions. There may be challenges to engage with, differing opinions and abilities or conflicts to address, all of which require you to demonstrate your burgeoning professional attributes and your newly developed skills. Remember, this is where you are assessed to determine whether you are fit to be in practice as a professional with people who are sometimes vulnerable for a number of reasons, which means you have to engage fully with the concept of professionalism and apply yourself fully to it. Although we recognise you are still learning, we have to engage with the overarching requirement to do no harm to those we work with, so you will have to remember this when in placement.

The professionals supporting you have all been where you are right now, so they know how you feel, what you might be worried about, what you need to be doing, and when things are not going smoothly. There are a number of processes around you to address all of the situations that arise in placement, and all of these are addressed in your placement handbook which will be pertinent to your chosen course and university. Consider, therefore, what placement might be like, remembering of course that no two placements are alike. We engage in our learning and development as individuals, so complete parity with our peers is improbable.

━━━━━━━ **ACTIVITY 2.4** ━━━━━━━

Reflection

When thinking about your placement, ask yourself:

- Is there anything I still want to know?
- Is there anything I do not understand?
- Do you feel more excited about going into placement (you might still feel nervous, but you will adjust)?
- Try to look for other information too and speak with your placement team at university.

Working Shifts

Though you are students, you are expected to work the same working pattern as all other staff. This may be starting a shift early morning, late in day, night shifts and weekends. Each student must work thirty-seven and a half hours a week. It is essential that you complete all allocated hours at work because successful completion of the course requires completion of practice hours set by your statutory professional body.

The placement team do consider the journey time to your placement but, on occasion, depending on where you live, you may have to travel further, so you need to consider this. The shifts you work will be identified by the practice area. On courses, other than social work, you may experience night duty from the first placement onwards. There are some differences between placements requirements on professional courses, so do please engage fully with your course handbook for more germane information.

Student Working Hours in Practice

The hours worked on placement (excluding breaks) must be recorded in your attendance record and signed by the relevant professional. It is your responsibility to maintain an accurate record of your completed placement hours. Any absence from placement must be recorded and you must inform the university. You may not undertake placement hours during academic learning weeks, as these are your theory hours. Attendance is required in placement at 100%.

Profession	Hours in placement	Days in placement
Nursing	2300	n/a
Midwifery	2300	n/a
ODP	2736	n/a
Paramedics	1640	n/a
Social Work	n/a	200 (approx. 9 am–5 pm)

You must consider and plan for childcare as you cannot take time off because of not having it in place. You have time to resolve it, so you need to plan ahead in good time. It will be far less stressful for you now than trying to get childcare in place as you go into placement. Finally, you also need to think about funding, as there are sometimes costs attached to placement and, while you might get a bursary payment, it is not guaranteed, so it cannot be relied upon.

━━━━━━━ **ACTIVITY 2.5** ━━━━━━━

Research and Reflection

1 In accordance with your area of interest, click on one of the links below:

How to survive your placement (nurses.co.uk) – In this video, a final year student, Eniola, shares her significant experiences from being on placement during her studies. It addresses some of the challenges and opportunities she experienced and it will help to demystify the practical element of the course, so that you have more confidence in your own placement.

What it's like being on PLACEMENT – Via's Student Vlog – YouTube – Via Pineda, a first-year student, shares her first day in placement to show you what it was really like. She discusses some of her concerns, such as not being able to implement her academic learning in practice and how these were resolved during the day.

Tips for Social Work Placements! – YouTube – In this video, Kayleigh Rose Evans offers some useful tips to social work students, such as developing good organisational skills, working with the pressure of successfully blending practical and academic learning, and meeting targets. She also discusses the need to look for opportunities, shadowing professionals and being proactive in placement.

What Happens When a Placement Is Going Wrong?

Case study 2.2

Mana

Mana has been missing days on placement. She thinks this is reasonable as she has childcare problems. The practice team contacts her academic assessor in the university. Having missed a number of days and not contacted the placement about her reasons for being absent, the practice team and education team organise a meeting with her. She does not turn up for the meeting and for the rest of the week. Her attendance to placement remained patchy and at an eventual meeting, an action plan was put in place. She continues to be absent on placement and at the end of her allocated placement, she fails the placement. She protests to the education team at the university of unfair treatment.

ACTIVITY 2.6

Critical Thinking and Reflection

How could this situation be prevented on placement?

How could Mana have managed her situation on placement?

What help and support could Mana have sought to ensure a positive outcome of her placement?

It could be argued that if Mana's childcare plans fell apart, then she had no choice but to care for her child. However, she has a professional responsibility towards her patients, the practice team and her colleagues. Importantly she has to complete her practice hours and professional competencies and values in order to meet the professional requirements for practice. Mana could have contacted the ward, in particular her practice supervisor and assessor to let them know her situation and reassured them that she has in place future child plans. She could have then met with the practice team, review her progress, re-set any goals and put an **action plan** in place to meet these goals. She could, alongside these actions, contact the named academic assessor in the university and her personal tutor to discuss her situation and seek advice and support of the possible options for achieving her practice hours and proficiencies and values. She could have sought help from the university support services regarding any childcare issues, financial matters and any other issues of concern.

It is essential that you engage in your learning in practice. In chapter 1, we discussed the important subject of student engagement in their learning, the benefits of you engaging and involving in your learning and tips for doing so. It is equally critical that you engage in your learning on placement as these same benefits apply.

Evidence of why some students fail to engage with their learning in practice point to a number of issues. The Open University summarised these (Mitchell, 2022, p. 3):

- a lack of insight, poor self-awareness and unresponsiveness to feedback
- a lack of interest, motivation, enthusiasm or commitment – not asking questions
- poor communication or interpersonal/interactional skills – insensitive interaction with patients
- frequently late or absent
- exhibit poor preparation and organisational skills
- preoccupation with personal issues – poor health, withdrawn, sad and tired
- poor professional behaviour/boundary issues
- either overconfident or underconfident
- lack of theoretical knowledge and skill, and provides limited evidence to support their learning
- avoidance of working with the mentor and changing shifts

Some of these factors will be familiar to students already on health and social care programmes. It is important for you as students seek support if you are experiencing challenges in practice. You can seek help from a variety of sources such as:

- practice supervisor/practice assessor/education facilitator
- academic assessor
- personal tutor
- student wellbeing team at the university
- wellbeing team in your placement organisation

It is better to seek help and get the support you need than to spend months on placement and find that you have failed the placement. Placement as we mentioned earlier can be challenging for students, so it is key that you talk with someone if you are experiencing any kind of difficulties.

Chapter Summary

The aim of this chapter is to help you gain an understanding of life in practice, often referred to as 'placement'. We discussed what constitutes practice and the challenges and opportunities of being in placement, including the different settings in which you will be practising. The preparations you will be given in university and in practice before you begin your placement have been detailed and should give you an insight into these two aspects of your course. We have outlined the role of your practice supervisor, assessor and academic assessor and set out the importance of regular communication with your practice and education team. The importance of ensuring your practice is successful through engaging in your learning, and tips for doing so in university are in Chapter 1 and tips for engaging in your placement are in this chapter. It is likely you may well encounter challenges in placement; thus we have set out strategies to help and support you.

3

What is Wellbeing?

Daniela Blumlein and
Annette Chowthi-Williams

NMC Standards of Proficiency for Registered Nurses (NMC, 2018)
Professional Standards Social Work England (2019)
Standards of Proficiency (HCPC, 2018)

Nursing & Midwifery Council

This chapter will address the following platforms and proficiencies:

1 Being an accountable professional
2 Promoting health and preventing ill health
6 Improving safety and quality of care

Social Work England

This chapter will address the following standards:

Standard 3: Be accountable for the quality of my practice and the decisions I make
Standard 4: Maintain my continuing professional development
Standard 5: Act safely and with professional integrity

Health and Care Professional Council

This chapter will address the following proficiencies:

1 be able to practise safely and effectively within their scope of practice
3 be able to maintain fitness to practise
4 be able to practise as an autonomous professional, exercising their own professional judgement
12 be able to assure the quality of their practice.

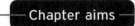

After reading this chapter, you will be able to:

- Understand the meaning of wellbeing for yourself and in a healthcare context.
- Describe situations and emotions that may lead to poor wellbeing.
- Reflect on your own wellbeing and how it affects your life.
- Develop strategies to maintain or enhance your wellbeing.

Introduction

In this chapter, we will explore the concept of wellbeing in general, in relation to staying well as a student on a health and social care course, and outline the benefits of wellbeing, in particular a high level of wellbeing. We will discuss factors that can positively or negatively impact on a person's wellbeing and address how this may apply to those in the caring professions. Healthcare workers often look after the wellbeing of their clients, patients and service users but may not focus on their own personal needs which may lead to them feeling stressed and less resilient. We will explore the strategies, tools and resources to support personal wellbeing and will offer some suggestions for self-care and maintaining or improving personal wellbeing for health and social care students, as well as signposting sources for further support.

What Does Wellbeing Mean?

The notion of wellbeing can mean different things to different people. The World Health Organization (WHO) (2020) suggests that wellbeing is more than simply not being physically sick or unwell. In their definition of positive mental health wellbeing, it is viewed as more than the absence of mental illness. It is about people believing their life is following the direction they wish it to go. Wellbeing comprises of a variety of factors, such as social, biological and psychological health (Engel, 1977), all of which have an impact on the way a person feels. Therefore, an individual may be free from disease but due to other issues in their life they may not feel a sense of being fully well which could have a negative impact on their quality of life. A person's sense of wellbeing could be affected by other life factors and determinants of health such as their housing situation, employment status, financial problems, peer pressure, loneliness and their access to healthcare and education (Linsley et al., 2011).

There are a variety of views, opinions and perspectives on the meaning of wellbeing. Ruggeri et al. (2020) research into wellbeing suggest that wellbeing is not just about being happy and satisfied with life and suggest a multidimensional measure of wellbeing might be more valuable for those in a policy making position. In their review of the literature on this subject, they outline the varying perspectives of wellbeing. Wellbeing seems to be interpreted as a mixture of positive feelings and managing well. In effect it is about feeling good, which translated into feeling happy, contented and being in control of one's life, one's future and having a sense of purpose. Not surprising, wellbeing is connected with a number of positive outcomes such as success in our personal and work life. They cite studies that suggest people whose wellbeing is elevated are not only more productive, resourceful, effective learners and have better relationships, but there are benefits to their physical health and generally they are more gratified with their lives.

Promoting wellbeing of staff and students is of benefit to everyone, including universities and the settings in which you will be practising your profession such as in acute or specialist hospitals, clinics, health centres, GP practices, in the homes of clients, patients and service users, in nursing and residential homes and in other settings. It can help to prevent long-term sickness and absence, as well as high staff turnover or attrition. Staying well and increasing resilience can help students to complete their course and become valued members of their chosen profession (Thomas, 2021).

━━━━━━━━ **ACTIVITY 3.1** ━━━━━━━━━━━━━━━━━

Reflection

Think about your wellbeing. What does wellbeing mean to you?

Make a note.

Think about the factors that contribute positively to your wellbeing.

Think about the factors that impact your wellbeing negatively.

Many countries across the world regularly measure the wellbeing of their population, and in the United Kingdom reports on the nation's wellbeing are published on a regular basis. The outcomes of these reports may be of great interest to you not only as a future health and social care professional but for you and your family because the report shows the state of wellbeing in various parts of the country in which you live. The latest personal wellbeing report in the United Kingdom covered a period from April 2020 to March 2021 and measured the nations' wellbeing using a number of indicators such as life satisfaction, happiness, anxiety and worthwhileness. The Office for National Statistics (ONS) (2021) measures wellbeing by asking people to give their views and opinions on a scale 0–10, how satisfied they are with their life. The evidence points to a worsening of the nation's wellbeing across all these areas. There was a deterioration in life satisfaction, anxiety has increased, happiness has declined and people feeling that their actions or activities are worthwhile has also dropped. However, this survey was over the COVID-19 pandemic and trends were similar in all countries in the United Kingdom.

━━━━━━━━━━ ACTIVITY 3.2 ━━━━━━━━━━

Research and Reflection

Explore the ONS report in the link below.

Read the section on personal wellbeing by local area.

Use the interactive map and explore the wellbeing in your local areas. https://www.ons.gov.uk/peoplepopulationandcommunity/wellbeing/bulletins/measuringnationalwellbeing/april2020tomarch2021

What Are the Benefits From Wellbeing?

There are many advantages to wellbeing and many studies have shown these benefits. Many organisations both in healthcare and in the business world now recognise the benefits of wellbeing to their employees and have programmes in place for supporting, improving and maintaining employees' wellbeing.

There is ample evidence on the positive effects of wellbeing and high wellbeing. Its impact is far and wide with positive effects on our health not just physical health but emotional, psychological, social and spiritual health. In a review of the evidence on subjective wellbeing and its impact on health, Diener et al. (2017) found that there is evidence that subjective wellbeing can influence our health and longevity. Healthcare organisations are now making such information public and available for their staff. The Royal Victoria Hospital (2022) details some of the benefits from wellbeing which are evidence-based.

- Feeling hopeful and experiencing positivity could lessen the risk of a heart attack
- People who are happy people live longer and may add another seven–eight years to your life
- Showing positive emotions ourselves can impact others positively
- High levels of wellbeing have benefits to our physical, mental and emotional health, for example:
- our ability to fight infection is higher
- our risk of some mental health complications is decreased
- we become more resilient
- protects the heart from coronary heart disease.

According to the Royal Victoria Hospital further evidence shows that people who experience higher levels of wellbeing tend to be:

- more involved in social activities and community groups
- environmentally responsible
- experiencing better family and social relationships at home
- more productive at work
- more likely to be working or studying full time
- more likely to recover quicker from a range of chronic diseases (e.g. diabetes) and
- in young people, higher levels of wellbeing significantly influence alcohol, tobacco and cannabis use.

https://5waystowellbeing.org.au/about-wellbeing/

Factors That Might Impact Your Wellbeing

Becoming a health and social care professional often includes a tight schedule of theory and clinical placements, and therefore can be very intense and demanding on the individual. In university students will have to complete a range of modules, meet essay deadlines, undertake exams and at times may need to re-take exams or re-submit an assignment. In the clinical settings, not only will you be working different shifts and with different teams and professionals but working in a clinical environment can be initially alienating and stressful for those new to the field. The day-to-day experience of caring and seeing patients, service users and clients in pain, discomfort or at the end of their life can lead to healthcare students becoming worried, upset and could ultimately lead to burnout.

Some studies have cited issues such as staff shortages, absenteeism, budget con-straints and interpersonal work relationships affecting those working in healthcare professions, and these factors add to the stress level that a student on clinical placement may experience (Wright et al., 2016). This may be because these aspects might impact the practice team supporting you in practice. If there is staff shortage and absenteeism, it will mean that the practice team's priority will be patient care.

These pressures combined with other factors such as personal financial worries, childcare issues, housing, relationship problems, tiredness and other personal commitments could lead to a student on such a course feeling like they are struggling, leading to them feeling stressed and in some situations, they may consider leaving the course (Mills et al., 2020). A further factor that has been affecting healthcare staff including students is the COVID-19 pandemic which has led to increased workloads, anxiety and stress for some in the profession and continues to be the case.

Case study 3.1

Amira

Amira is studying currently in her first year of her course. She has to complete an essay in the next week and has just started her first placement on a busy surgical ward. She has two children, twins, who are four years old, and she shares childcare responsibilities with her boyfriend Ross.

Recently, Ross and Amira have been arguing a lot and he has started staying at his friend's house and has been not there some mornings to look after the children and Amira had to miss time on her placement. Amira stays up most of the night waiting for Ross as she is very worried and cannot sleep easily. She has not had time to work on her essay and has had headaches most days as well as feeling anxious and very sad. Her practice assessor has contacted the university to raise concerns about her attendance and has called a meeting to discuss an action plan with Amira and her Academic Assessor. Amira is frightened that she will not pass her placement.

ACTIVITY 3.3

Research and Reflection

What are the issues impacting on Amira's wellbeing and how may they affect her nursing course?

What advice would you give Amira if she were your classmate?

Strategies to Improve Your Own Wellbeing

Students in health and social care undertaking a programme of study to become a qualified professional do have codes of conduct by which they have to practice. Should they not abide by their respective codes, they will face disciplinary procedure and in some case be removed from the profession. However, these codes of conduct also advise on the importance of prioritising one's own health and wellbeing and instruct professionals on their responsibility for ensuring their health and wellbeing in order to practice safely and effectively. Thus, students must inform placement and the university if they are unwell and seek help to ensure they are fit to carry out their responsibilities. Students therefore should not carry on with the course or placements as they may put service user, patients and clients at risk due to their own poor health or wellbeing. This does not mean a student must leave the course; however, they must seek support and treatment and work with their respective university to ensure they can return to the course only when they are ready. Often, there is no need to step off the course or to take sick leave, as often the way a person feels can be managed by practising self-care and increasing resilience.

There are strategies and resources a healthcare student could utilise to improve or maintain their own wellbeing.

- Recognising early on when you become stressed and exhausted is very important.
- Knowing that you can take simple steps to regain strength and avoid it becoming a bigger issue.
- By prioritising one's own wellbeing and physical and mental health, you are ensuring that you are fit to look after service users, patients and clients; thus it could be asserted that by looking after yourself, you are protecting your clients.
- It may seem logical that when someone is studying for a course, that it is best to only concentrate on the learning and neglect socialising or hobbies; however, aim for balance and do things that help you relax and feel good about yourself.
- You may think it's best to limit recreational activities during your time on a course; however, it is not beneficial in the long term and may lead to burnout at a later stage.
- Finding a healthy balance between studying and relaxing is the best way to achieve success.

ACTIVITY 3.4

Reflection

It is Friday evening, and you had a very busy week at university.
List four things you may do to relax and switch off.

You may have mentioned activities such as meeting friends, watching TV, going for a walk, cuddling with a pet or playing football. Some of the things you may have mentioned in the above activity may be very positive. However, sometimes individuals may also engage in behaviours that may feel stress relieving at the time but could have a negative effect in the long term. These coping strategies may include drinking too much alcohol to relax or taking recreational drugs or engaging in other risky behaviours. It is important that you recognise which strategies on improving wellbeing are positive and which could lead to you feeling worse. Focus on those that make you feel better in the long-term rather than short-term fixes such as drinking or shopping. If you feel you are struggling to give up unhelpful behaviours, it may be beneficial to speak to a friend, your personal tutor, your GP or a counsellor.

Practising self-care and improving wellbeing could consist of something as simple as taking a long bath or listening to calming music and reading a book. Mills et al. (2020) researched the experiences of undergraduate nursing students, and some of the strategies students used to deal with stress and fatigue included:

- physical exercise
- getting enough sleep
- eating healthily
- spending time in nature

Having a good social support network, such as family and friends or joining a sports club, as often face-to-face interaction is more valuable than online networking. It is easy to fall into a habit of spending lots of time scrolling through social networking sites; however, this may not always help you to feel relaxed, so try to set a time limit for online activity.

━━━━━━━━━━ **ACTIVITY 3.5** ━━━━━━━━━━

Research and Reflection

Make a list of all the social network websites you visited today and estimate how long you spend doing this.

How did you feel afterwards?

What feelings did you experience during the time you spend scrolling?

Some of your answers may have included feeling happy to connect with family members and friends and seeing how they are doing or reading an interesting post on a subject that interests you. You may have even visited a website that promotes relaxation and wellbeing, and it is possible that you felt better and positive after doing this. However, you may have also answered that you spend long periods simply scrolling through social media posts that were not interesting to you, or even upset you. Perhaps you felt that other people lead a more interesting life compared to yours or you felt triggered or reminded of something negative in your past by something someone posted. It is also possible that your self-esteem may have been affected by seeing photoshopped images of celebrities and you felt pressurised to live up to those standards. If you mentioned some of the latter issues, then it may be that you could benefit from limiting your time online and engaging in more real-life activities.

It is also important to remember that social media posts are aimed at presenting a person's best version of themselves, so it is not realistic to try and achieve a lifestyle that is portrayed online in most cases. You could try to stay off the internet for a day or a weekend and see if your wellbeing improves after a period of 'digital detoxing'.

At times, it can be hard to focus your thoughts and attention on something, especially when you feel tired or stressed.

- A useful technique for relaxation and focus is practising mindfulness, which Cottrell (2018) likens to pressing the pause button and taking time to notice the here and now.
- Mindfulness can be seen as a tool to take time out and to reclaim one's thoughts.
- This ancient technique can be used to help increase wellbeing, empathy, concentration, as well as lower stress levels and anxiety.
- It can also be a positive action to take before an exam, writing an essay or when things are very stressful on a clinical placement.
- In the modern world individuals are constantly subject to numerous stimuli such as noise and social media, which can lead to feelings of exhaustion and feeling like things are getting too much.
- Initially, a person may only practice mindfulness for a short period, such as a few minutes, while more experienced practitioners of the technique may take much longer.

McVeigh et al. (2015) carried out a research study on how mindfulness can benefit student nurses and found that some students reported they found the practice useful and that it enhanced their self-care. However, not everybody enjoyed mindfulness, so it may not suit everyone, and it is something that needs to be decided on a personal level. If you are interested in trying mindfulness for yourself, you can utilise a multitude of tools such as books, websites and apps that can help you learn the technique, or you may prefer to enrol on a face-to-face mindfulness class. Mindfulness can involve meditation or simply noticing what is going on in your surroundings, such as listening to sounds you can hear. You may start to notice thought patterns that come and go or focus on your breathing (Cottrell, 2018).

More Sources of Support

The previous section has discussed a variety of approaches and strategies that can be used to improve a person's wellbeing and prioritise self-care. However, if a student on a health and social care course feels that they are not able to address a problem that affects their wellbeing by themselves, there are more sources of support that can be accessed:

- universities and other education providers often have a department that can provide advice on topics such as wellbeing, additional learning needs and mental health support.
- these services are free of charge and confidential, and details of how to gain access to them can often be found on an organisation's website or via student services.

- a further resource will be your personal tutor or your course leader, who can also offer pastoral care and talk to you about your worries.
- they can also signpost you to departments that can provide further support. For example, you may raise a concern about your essay writing skills with your personal tutor and they may refer you to your education provider's learning and skill development department.

Additionally, your student union representative will be able to listen to your worries and try to help you find support, as well as acting as a mediator if there are any problems with your education provider. Student unions often organise days out and events that help you to make new friends on your course or to increase wellbeing, so it is always a good idea to look out for what is on offer. Perhaps you have a special skill that others may enjoy learning?

- you could liaise with the student union to set up a group or society to get others involved and this could help your peers to relax and learn something new, while also increasing your self-esteem and wellbeing.
- peer support from your classmates is also a valuable resource to increase wellbeing.
- try to share your experiences on the course that you are studying with others in safe environment, and you may learn that what you are experiencing is also what others are going through.
- talking to someone you trust can help you to feel well and increase your social circle.
- if you need support while on a clinical placement, you should seek support and guidance from your practice or the academic team, who will be able to help you reflect on new experiences and maximise your learning.
- if you feel that you may need more urgent support, you should contact your GP without delay and arrange an appointment.
- your university/education provider has many sources of help, so please remember to ask for help and do not suffer in silence.

━━━━━━━ **ACTIVITY 3.6** ━━━━━━━

Research and Reflection

Rashid has so far enjoyed his course very much. He achieved excellent grades in the first year, but in the second year, he is not doing so well. He has not passed his last two exams and needs to repeat them. Rashid is a carer for his mother who has dementia and lives with him. Rashid feel like everything is going wrong for him at the moment and is considering leaving his course. He has been crying a lot and has not gone to see his friends at the tennis club recently.

Make a list of sources of support Rashid could access to help him get back on track with his studies and to improve his wellbeing.

The NHS (2019) advises five steps to mental wellbeing. They set actions that people should undertake and activities to stay away from.

Helpful actions to undertake are as follows:

- Connect with others
- Be physically active
- Learn new skills
- Give to others
- Pay attention to the present moment

Actions to keep away from are as follows:

- Try not to depend on social media for relationships.
- Try not to exercise and undertake activities that will bring you pain or are unenjoyable.
- If you wish to learn a new skill, ensure you will enjoy it.

https://www.nhs.uk/mental-health/self-help/guides-tools-and-activities/five-steps-to-mental-wellbeing/

The international bestseller author Adriana Huffington in her book *Thrive* suggests three simple steps we can all take to improve our wellbeing.

- Get 30 minutes more sleep. Take short nap during the day or get to bed a little earlier.
- Move your body; walk, run, stretch, do yoga, dance. Just move. Anytime.
- Introduce five minutes of meditation into your day and build up to 15 or 20 minutes a day.

Most of these strategies and tools are all easily accessible and we have provided the links to some of these. It is essential as future health and social care student that you do practice self-care. It is a professional responsibility not to put your patients, service users and clients at risk of any harm.

Chapter Summary

This chapter discussed wellbeing and how it relates to students on a health and social care course. The concept of wellbeing was explored from a number of perspectives and in general there is agreement on the idea of wellbeing. The sense of high wellbeing can have a positive outcome on our holistic health and our feeling of happiness and life satisfaction. Issues that can affect wellbeing were discussed and a range of factors were identified that can impact our wellbeing. We explored the many strategies for support and self-care available for health and social care students. We also considered additional support. These activities are aimed at helping students to develop their skills and to utilise what they have learned in this chapter.

4

Creating Emotional and Mental Balance

Janet Goddard, Regina Holley and Raquel Marta

NMC Standards of Proficiency for Registered Nurses (NMC, 2018)
Professional Standards Social Work England (2019)
Standards of Proficiency (HCPC, 2018)

Nursing & Midwifery Council

This chapter will address the following platforms and proficiencies:

1 Being an accountable professional
2 Promoting health and preventing ill health
3 Assessing needs and planning care
4 Providing and evaluating care
7 Coordinating care

Social Work England

This chapter will address the following standards:

Standard 1: Promote the rights, strengths and wellbeing of people, families and communities
Standard 2: Establish and maintain the trust and confidence of people
Standard 3: Be accountable for the quality of my practice and the decisions I make
Standard 4: Maintain my continuing professional development

Health and Care Professional Council

This chapter will address the following proficiencies:

1   be able to practise safely and effectively within their scope of practice
3   be able to maintain fitness to practise
4   be able to practise as an autonomous professional, exercising their own professional judgement
8   be able to communicate effectively
9   be able to work appropriately with others
11   be able to reflect on and review practice
12   be able to assure the quality of their practice
14   be able to draw on appropriate knowledge and skills to inform practice

---

Chapter aims

After reading this chapter, you will be able to:

* Recognise the role of the mind and different types of emotion and understand how they might impact you.
* Be able to reflect on how you are feeling, using one or more emotions.
* Identify ways in which you might deal with your emotions before reacting to other people.
* Demonstrate an awareness of emotional wellbeing and its impact on you.

Introduction

Our mind, consciousness and emotions are linked, and it is important to understand these connections. In this chapter, we will begin by exploring the nature of the mind and how it is embodied in the interactions we have with others and the environment. The discussion goes on to identify nurturing mind strategies to cultivate wellbeing and it will help you to develop a robust understanding of emotions and their impact on behaviour and responses to situations. In the final part of the chapter, we will explore the workings of the mind and emotion and consider strategies to optimise positive wellbeing and limit maladaptive emotional responses, particularly in the social setting of the workplace. We will invite you to reflect on your own emotional resources and to begin to consider strategies to strengthen them. We will have activities to engage with and scenarios to underpin your engagement with critical thinking, which is a skill that will serve you well on your professional course.

The Importance of Mind

Imagine that your mind lives inside a backpack and that you open the backpack to look inside at its contents. What would you find? Images. An enormous diversity of images. Images that you create, images that you combine, imagines that you idealise. These are the images of reality – the landscapes you see, the sounds you listen to, the ideas you imagine, the projects you anticipate, the objects you touch, the events you experience, the aspirations you have – resulting from an intrinsic body/mind connection in interaction with the world that surround us, thus, always in motion.

As Damasio (2018) underlines, in normal circumstances, when we are aware and alert, the images that flow through our mind have one perspective only: our own. We recognise ourselves as owning the mental experiences we are exposed to. Each one of us appreciates that specific mental state accordantly with different perspectives: mine/yours.

Traditionally, the mind has been associated with the linear associations performed in the brain activity, but recent research has brought into discussion the notion that the mind is both embodied and relational (Siegel, 2020). This means that, together, mind, body and features of our interpersonal relationships and of the environments in which we live regulate both energy and information flow. To better understand the embodiment and the relational nature of mind consider, for example, how do you think and feel both individually and when in a group or in a community: the interpersonal experiences that you might have, while in a group/community influence how your mind processes the images information and how it works. This means that your internal mental experience – your sense of knowing, of imagining and being aware – is enriched and challenged by the subjective nature of interactions that occur between you and others, and between you and the environment.

Is the Mind Conscient?

Mind and consciousness, as Damasio alerts, 'are not synonymous' (Damasio, 2021, p. 135). Consciousness is a distinctive and subjective state of mind that allows us to integrate the experiences we are exposed to. Let us go back to the images in your backpack: without conscience all these images will be meaningless, deprived from any type of value. The conscience is what makes the mental experiences possible: think of everything you learn, remember, manipulate or, as Koch (2018, p. S9) illustrates: 'It is the tune stuck in your head, the sweetness of chocolate mousse, the throbbing pain of a toothache, the fierce love for your child and the bitter knowledge that eventually all feelings will end'. Our consciousness involves, then, a variety of distinctive experiences that imply more than mental images, as it also includes conscious experiences that arise from real sensations, feelings and experiences.

Creating Wellbeing: Conscious Mind Training What Can You Do?

Beyond the provision of the professional support available, you play a core role in developing awareness, strategies and promoting a positive state of mental wellbeing for yourself. Therefore, the choice to train your mind is, naturally, sensitive to your own life experience, your own cultural, social, spiritual and environmental dynamics. Additionally, as an upcoming professional, one of the major challenges ahead is also connecting yourself to the continuously changing social, political, educational and environmental conditions in relation to your future everyday professional practice. As different kinds of experiences shape the way your mind works, we share below different suggestions:

- ***Delve yourself into a world of imagination and creativity***
  Imagination and creativity are skills that you would aim to understand and develop to face the unpredictability and complexity of life. Embedded in imagination, creativity is, *per se*, a stimulant for the mind allowing different ways of thinking and embracing different perspectives. Whether you are actively engaged with an art activity (e.g., chorus), visiting a museum, finding shapes in the cloud's movements, or simply ingeniously expanding yourself while dancing in your living room, you are creating elements of originality and expressiveness. Creativity has a significant impact on the health and wellbeing of each one of us and results from a recent large study (BBC, 2019) highlighted 3 ways you can actively use it:

  - As a distraction tool – so we can use creativity, inspiration and imagination to avoid stress.
  - As a contemplation tool – using creativity to give us the space to think and re-evaluate problems in our lives and make plans for resolving them.
  - As a means of growth and self-development to face challenges by building up and reinforcing our self-esteem and self-confidence. It is important to keep in mind, then, that engaging in imaginative and creative activities have long-term benefits, including handling your own mood and boosting your overall wellbeing, allowing your mind a healthy gateway (APPGAHW, 2017; BBC, 2019).

- *Develop mindful awareness*

  Studies on the physical and mental health benefits of mindfulness have been growing for the past two decades; yet, as noted by Smith et al. (2017), a review on the existent literature on mindfulness and meditation highlighted there is still no consensual definition or common understanding of its impact. The Oxford Mindfulness Centre defines mindfulness as an intrinsic aptitude transversal to all human beings, a state of mind that allows us to focus in the moment, free from any judgemental chains; it is like a quiet inner exploration aligned with the structure of your consciousness. Some of the most ancient mindful practices are yoga and meditation, but there are so many more that you can explore from breathing exercises to mindful seeing, to find the best mindful practice for you.

  While debates around mindfulness definition and mindful awareness practices continue, there are some benefits already consensually identified (Smith et al., 2017):

  - Intensification of resilience to stress.
  - Improvement in attention focus, reducing mind-wandering and, consequently, stimulating concentration and problem-solving skills development.
  - Self-compassion and compassion behaviours increase.
  - Positive impact in mental health.
  - Reduces bias and, thus, promotes tolerance.
  - Beneficial to relationships, as mindfulness could have a positive impact on your relationships.The beauty of mindful practice is that it can be applied to everyday life events or routines while embracing one's wellbeing.

- *Cultivate the sense of gratitude*

  An increasing body of research is beginning to study how gratitude improves different features of our life and how it contributes to a healthy mind (Allen, 2018; Short, 2021). As Allen (2018) points out, nurturing the practice of gratitude inspires us to value what is good in our live, to develop new relationships and enrich the existent ones. Gratitude meaning can vary from person to person, but overtime, it has been recognised and conceptualised as 'an emotion, an attitude, a moral virtue, a habit, a personality trait or a coping response' (Short, 2021, p. 130). Understood in these terms, the experience of gratitude embraces different features of our personality development (individual factors) and the way we live the emotional, the cultural, the social, the religious dimensions of our life (social factors). Generated by value, gratitude can be seen as an integrated multi-value practice involving a range of behaviours and actions that shape the person we are and the relationships we have with others with a variety of beneficial outcomes (Allen, 2018; Short, 2021) such as:

- Increase of the energy levels, the enthusiasm and determination.
- A real sense of happiness, joy and satisfaction. Values the feeling of self-worth.
- Stimulates emotional intelligence development.
- Fuels the conscious mind in the search for opportunities of development.
- Refines cognitive skills such as creativity and fosters social connections.
- Development of resilience mechanisms and associated improvement of mental health.Engaging and cultivating gratitude practices is simple and, just like the mindful practices, can be incorporated in our daily life.

━━━━━━━ **ACTIVITY 4.1** ━━━━━━━

Reflection and Practice

Choose one of the following exercises:

1 Go for a walk by the streets of your city or town. Pay attention to the details, look for an open-air art gallery or the unrestricted and diverse street art also known as graffiti and appreciate it. Perhaps you will identify, and question embedded political statements, perhaps you will be enchanted by the aesthetic of a mural. The possibilities are immense.
2 Select a place that makes you feel good, either indoors or outdoors. Focus on your breathing and calmly start developing an awareness of the length and depth of each breath in and out. Start a 10-minute timer and initiate controlled inhaling through your nose and exhaling through your mouth. Make sure you feel the deepness of your breathing into your core. Find your own exercise pace and repeat it regularly.
3 Write a short thank you note for yourself or for a person that you like to nurture. Expressing appreciation will make you both happier. Try to do it recurrently.

Emotions

Emotions cover aspects of how we feel, they are subjective and transient, fluid or changing and we might change our emotional 'state' throughout the day depending on what we are doing. So, what do we really understand when we think of emotion, do we think of only one feeling, or do we think of a range of feelings from vague to deep? When we speak of feeling happy, sad, afraid, angry, nervous, tearful or excited, what we are doing is describing our emotional state (Tantam, 2014). We sometimes feel two or more emotions, so we might feel happy and excited, or tearful and afraid, or even happy and tearful at the same time. Sometimes our emotions are identifiers of our internal state, but other times they are in response to an external factor (Barrett, 2018). So, we might feel nervous if we are waiting for a grade for a paper we have submitted and then happy or sad depending on whether we passed the assessment or not. We can also hide our feelings, so we might show the world a different picture to how we really feel (Satpute et al., 2016), for example, we might look happy when we are feeling quite sad (Barrett, 2018). We know, therefore, that emotions trigger or underpin behavioural, hormonal, somatic or pathological, and neurochemical reactions, which we refer to as 'expressions of emotion' (Zach & Gogolla, 2021).

ACTIVITY 4.2

How Do You Feel Right Now?

Describe how you feel. Are you feeling a mix of emotions, or is one emotion more powerful than the other?

Image Source - (GDJ) https://openclipart.org/detail/222289/bright-idea

---

The chances are that you considered only a few emotions, but research proposes there are 27 distinct categories, which are bridged by continuous gradients (Cowen & Keltner, 2017). While there has been a significant body of research on emotions, we tend instead to think of them from an automatous, perfunctory perspective, focusing on our physiological, psychological, cognitive or as a behavioural response to a specific experience or event, but emotions can be complex and create within us a psychophysiological response; so, we might feel angry or upset and our heart may feel as if it is racing where we experience a blend of an emotional and physical response to something (Nagoski, 2020), but we can also experience the same physiological response to love or excitement which means our physical response to situations is only a part of our reaction and our psychological response is another. We can also consider the positive aspect of this union between the mental and physical response to something; so, before we sit an exam, we might naturally feel nervous or anxious. This natural feeling is releasing cortisol and adrenaline, which are both stress hormones, into our body which will allow us to be ready for the challenge of the exam (Partridge, 2020). So, when you start to feel anxious and jittery, try to remember that this is normal and is your body and mind preparing you for the task in front of you.

Case study 4.1

Bob

Bob is coming to the end of the first semester and about to sit his assessments. When he joined the university, he was very concerned he would not be able to keep up with the work and pass the assessments. Bob failed one paper at college and can remember how upset he was when he saw his grade. He now keeps remembering how he felt, and although he is worried about all of the assessments, he is particularly worried about an upcoming exam which is making him feel very stressed and anxious.

━━━━━ **ACTIVITY 4.3** ━━━━━

Critical Thinking

Read the scenario above and think about Bob's situation.

Can you understand how he is feeling?

What would you advise him to do?

Think about Bob's experience when he failed his assessment at college. Think about yourself. Do you have any similar concerns? What are they? Can you put them into simple words to explain them to another person? What might help you to feel less stressed or anxious?

Make a note of how you might address any concerns around your studies and assessments as this will allow you to really think about how you are feeling and consider what events make you feel more anxious. Think also of what you could do to support yourself or help others support you if the concerns feel overwhelming as this will allow you to be proactive and seek out the support you might need.

The effect of emotions on our body can be significant but serve different purposes; for example, you may find that you have heard of the 'fight or flight' response to stimuli, which is involved in self-preservation (Quick & Spielberger, 1994) but it might be that you have less awareness of how unresolved emotional responses can affect our day-to-day functioning. McGonigal (2015) proposes that stress can also be a force of good, for change, and for development; so instead of trying to avoid addressing a situation, or denying there is a problem, or starting to withdraw from your studies, recognise that these are not helpful responses as you may end up facing a bigger problem later. So, what can you do to address it? See below (Figure 4.1):

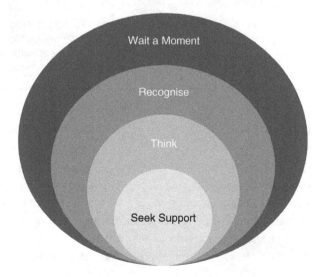

Figure 4.1 Steps in positive emotional stress management

i. **Wait a moment**

This is important because, sometimes, we react immediately to something and create a different problem for ourselves, so stopping before reacting can allow us to think it through a little more clearly.

ii. **Recognise**

It is important to recognise your feelings and think about why something is affecting you so much, for example, does it make you remember something that happened previously, or has your day not started well and the issue that occurred made it worse. It is fine for you to feel upset by something, but it is important to not make someone else responsible for something they have no knowledge of.

iii. **Think**

Now that you are in the 'thinking' phase, points for consideration might be

- What is the issue for you?
- How are you feeling?
- What could be the outcome of you reacting?
- What is another way to deal with the issue?
- What can you do for yourself to make you feel better?

iv. **Seek Support**

- What support might you need?
- How might you access it?
- Who can you speak with?

━━━━━━━ ACTIVITY **4.4** ━━━━━━━

Reflection

Go back to Case Study 4.1 and remind yourself of Bob's situation.

Think about making a plan to help prevent any anxiety or stress around your own assessments. What might you include in it? Your plan could include things like pre-planning, writing support, help with proofreading, or help with referencing. Remember it is your plan, personal and bespoke for you, so focus only on what you need.

Mind and Emotion

One of our uniquely human qualities is the ability to think and reflect on experiences in any situation. The thinking we apply to our experiences can affect our emotional responses. Likewise, our emotions can affect our thinking (Barrett, 2018). This synergistic relationship can be beneficial in that it allows us to have a holistic sense of our experiences, which allows us to learn from them, achieve personal growth, and move on. However, the opposite can also be the case. Negative thoughts, often stemming from previous experiences, can infiltrate our emotions and cause us to have maladaptive responses in our environment.

Until recently, the popular belief was that our emotional experiences influence our thinking. However, recent research by Barrett (2018) suggests that it is our brain that uses its predictive power to construct our emotions. This suggests that we have more control over our emotions than we think we do.

The Mind and the Emotion in Context

The work of health and social care professionals involves a high level of physical and emotional interaction with patients, clients, service users and between staff. Challenges in the health and social care environment contribute to staff stress and burnout (Kings Fund, 2018) which according to Hagemeister and Volmer (2018) can promote social conflict in the workplace; so how do we resolve this? Most people are able to manage their emotions, but some use 'Display Rules' defined as the expression of positive emotions while masking negative emotions (Fasbinder, Shidler, & Caboral-Stevens, 2020, p. 118). This type of adaptive approach to emotional stress leads to longer-term negative wellbeing consequences and contributes to stress, burnout and a range of physical and mental health problems which calls for an emotional regulation.

The ability to regulate emotions is key to avoiding negative consequences for personal and professional wellbeing and to optimally support patients and clients. Emotional regulation is a learned process and involves the ability to identify your emotion, the meaning the emotion has for you and how you experience and express the emotion. It allows us to recognise and find alternative responses to the beliefs we have created about ourselves, others and our surroundings, but because we are not born with emotional regulation, it needs to be developed and this requires self-work and self-care.

Gross (2015), who conducted early research in this area, identified reappraisal and suppression as commonly used approaches to emotion regulation. While reappraisal is about cognitively reframing a negative situation in a positive light in order to change the negative emotional impact, suppression is about modifying your response to the situation, sometimes by inhibiting your natural response. Kelly et al. (2018) argues that both strategies are successful in reducing the negative impact of a situation; but suppression is seen as a more maladaptive approach that can lead to the return of negative emotional responses (Brockman et al., 2016).

Resilience Building and Emotional Regulation

Emotion-driven thinking is a component of our emotional responses (McKay, Fanning, & Zurita, 2011) and is the way our mind works to give meaning to a situation. McKay and colleagues propose that our cognitive responses can be divided into predicting what might happen as a result of a situation or making a judgement. They argue that while predictions can prepare us for a future event, they can also create stress and anxiety about something that may never happen.

Judgement tends to be negative about the subject of the situation and this can trigger further negative emotions. If you are the object of the situation, then judging yourself using negative ruminating thoughts can leave you feeling sad or depressed. When other people are the object and we judge them negatively, this can create feelings of anger and resentment and cause rifts in social relationships (Arimitsu, 2015). A healthy way to manage our reactions is to use emotional regulation strategies.

We often use emotionally driven thoughts to create beliefs about ourselves, others and our surroundings. McKay, Fanning, and Zurita (2011) suggest dividing these thoughts into two categories, predicting and judgement.

- Predicting what could happen. These are the 'what-if' questions we ask ourselves when we think about what might happen in a situation. These predictions tend to be negatively biased. The problem with this kind of thinking is that you can catastrophise a situation and project yourself down a 'rabbit hole'. For example: 'What if I fail the assignment?' 'I will be removed from the course,' 'I will be so ashamed'. 'My family will be very disappointed in me' and so on.

- Judgement of the incident and the people involved. This is how we evaluate and draw conclusions about ourselves, others and the situation. This type of thinking is usually based on the positive or negative emotions we generate about ourselves, others and the situation. For example, you may get a poor grade on an assignment, and one way to understand this is to assess the situation and the people involved, including yourself. For example, 'the assignment guidelines were very confusing', 'the tutor did not explain things well', 'I am just not smart enough to become a social work/nursing student'.

Prediction and judgement responses are not without history and consequences. We base our judgements on past experiences, often in our social circle of family, friends or founded on our upbringing. These emotionally based thoughts can lead to feelings of sadness, depression and anger which, if left unchecked, can lead to increased feelings of worthlessness, decreased self-esteem and a lack of self-confidence. This can result in poor decision making.

━━━━━━━━━━━ **ACTIVITY 4.5** ━━━━━━━━━━━

Reflection

Reflect on a situation where your thoughts, driven by your emotions, led you down a 'rabbit hole'. What alternative thoughts could you have had to avoid catastrophising a situation?

━━━━━━━━━━━━ **ACTIVITY 4.6** ━━━━━━━━━━━━

Reflection

Reflect on an incident where you came to a conclusion about yourself, others and the situation related to the incident.

Reflect on your thoughts at the time. It helps if you write them down.

Do you still believe that thought?

Case study 4.2

Shirley

Shirley was asked to call a relative to pick up her partner from the unit. She knows this is an easy task, but it is her first time calling a relative and she is keen to get it right. She writes down the instructions and is given the phone number. Before she could make the call, Shirley was asked to help her colleague. This took longer than she expected, and she realises that she is now late with the call. Shirley hurriedly makes a phone call but because she is nervous, she forgets that the instructions are in her bag.

When a person answers the phone, Shirley starts right away and gives all the details until the person interrupts her to say that her partner came home yesterday. Shirley checks the number she was given and finds that she was given another person's number. She apologises and quickly hangs up the phone. She worries that she may have compromised a patient's confidentiality.

━━━━━━━━━━━━ **ACTIVITY 4.7** ━━━━━━━━━━━━

Critical Thinking

Read the scenario above and think about Shirley's situation.

- What might Shirley be feeling and how might these feelings affect her thinking?
- What prediction might Shirley make based on the situation?
- What judgement might Shirley make based on the situation?

One of the first steps in understanding how and why we react to the different situations we encounter is to understand the internal and external influences on those reactions. Manstead (2005) emphasises the role of the social environment in influencing our emotional responses and expression. Zych and Gogolla (2021) argue that there is a mutual relationship between the social environment and our reactions and the meaning we give to our experiences.

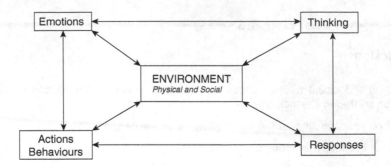

Figure 4.2 Graphic representation of the mutual correlations between mind, emotion and the environment

The following diagram provides a visual framework that illustrates the synergic nature of the interaction between our mind, emotion and the environment (Figure 4.2).

Our mind and emotions work together to form responses and form experiences. This can have positive and negative influences on how we interact with our social environment. Our ability to function within the social environment in the workplace requires us to be able to regulate our emotions. Being aware of how to evaluate and think about a situation can be the first step in regulating our response which can bring about a more positive outcome for us.

Chapter Summary

We started this chapter by introducing the importance of understanding how our mind works and how our mental wellbeing also correlates with specific states of mind. We used several examples to illustrate how you can develop mind training strategies to promote your wellbeing. This was followed by the discussion of role and effect of emotions. Even though our emotional state is formed from a complex set of processes that were not explored in depth, we hope it has become clear to you that emotions are a central part of the process that generates a certain state of mind in a specific context; and that they are at the core of internal and interpersonal processes that create the subjective experience of yourself and the world. Being able to regulate your mind will help you to manage your emotions which will enable you to function optimally in the health and social care spaces. Throughout this book, there are links and further advice to do with managing your emotions and stress, so do read it but also keep it with you as you can refer back to it when you need to.

5

Managing Own and Other's Emotions in Practice

Kate Nash and Cathy Rowan

Professional Standards of Proficiency used to Support this Chapter
NMC Standards of Proficiency for Registered Nurses (NMC, 2018)
Professional Standards Social Work England (2019)
Standards of Proficiency (HCPC, 2018)

Nursing & Midwifery Council

This chapter will address the following platforms and proficiencies:

1 Being an accountable professional.
2 Promoting health and preventing ill health.
5 Leading and managing nursing care and working in teams.

Social Work England

This chapter will address the following standards:

Standard 1: Promote the rights, strengths and wellbeing of people, families and
communities
Standard 3: Be accountable for the quality of my practice and the decisions I make
Standard 4: Maintain my continuing professional development
Standard 5: Act safely and with professional integrity

Health and Care Professional Council

This chapter will address the following proficiencies:

3   be able to maintain fitness to practise
4   be able to practise as an autonomous professional, exercising their own professional
judgement
8   be able to communicate effectively
9   be able to work appropriately with others
11 be able to reflect on and review practice
12 be able to assure the quality of their practice
14 be able to draw on appropriate knowledge and skills to inform practice

---

Chapter aims

After reading this chapter, you will be able to:

- Understand the nature of caring within a healthcare context.
- Understand the emotions you might encounter and experience within clinical practice.
- Reflect upon your own emotional responses and consider how you can respond in a
professional way to different situations.
- Develop appropriate supportive strategies to manage your emotions and those of others.

Introduction

We will begin in this chapter with exploring the nature of caring and what it means to
you. We will consider the impact of the emotions that may be involved with caring
and encourage you to reflect upon your emotional responses to help you understand
your emotions and recognise how they might influence your own wellbeing. We will
explore how your emotions might also influence your professional behaviour and the

care you provide within practice. On an individual basis, your emotional responses will be different depending on your background, circumstances, personality and previous experiences. We will consider various strategies that may be used to help you manage your emotions in a professional context. Various activities and case studies will be used to support the discussion throughout this chapter.

The Nature of Caring and Emotions Within a Healthcare Context

Caring is at the heart of the healthcare professional's role and embedded within our actions. It is important to be aware of the emotional components of caring to enable you to provide compassionate care. Compassion has been described as intelligent kindness and providing care through relationships with others that are based on empathy, respect and dignity (NHS England, 2014). The NHS Constitution sets out the key principles that guide the NHS in all it does which are underpinned by core values which include compassion.

The NHS Constitution. (2021). Available https://www.gov.uk/government/publications/the-nhs-constitution-for-england/the-nhs-constitution-for-england

Compassion

We ensure that compassion is central to the care we provide and respond with humanity and kindness to each person's pain, distress, anxiety or need. We search for the things we can do, however small, to give comfort and relieve suffering. We find time for patients, their families and carers, as well as those we work alongside. We do not wait to be asked, because we care. The provision of care and compassion within a healthcare context can be emotionally demanding. Emotional labour may be described as the devaluing of emotions arising from work and alienation from one's own feelings within the workplace (Traynor, 2017). The emotional work of nursing is a great influence on practitioner's wellbeing which has previously been overlooked in practice (Smith, 2012). Thus, nurses have often been expected to manage their personal emotions in isolation and to remain calm in the face of critical illness in patients or create a calm exterior to colleagues in stressful situations (Kirk, 2021). The emotions health professionals might experience within the workplace may become diminished or hidden to prioritise the immediate needs of the patient and family.

Evidence of the impact of emotional work on healthcare practitioners

There is ample evidence of the impact of emotional work on healthcare professional. The demands of healthcare are ever expanding. As a healthcare professional you will be providing care for people when they are at their most vulnerable. Caring for people during challenging life moments can be emotionally demanding for you and others. Working long hours and varied shift patterns may increase symptoms of stress and fatigue in those working within a hospital setting (Ball et al., 2014). Healthcare professionals can suffer from symptoms such as stress, burnout and compassion fatigue because of the emotional work of caring. Burnout is described as a feeling of detachment, lack of personal accomplishment and emotional exhaustion.

Professor Billie Hunter has made a significant contribution to our knowledge about the emotional work of midwifery and has proposed that an emotion management continuum exists as practitioners juggle the demands of daily practice – with one end of the continuum representing the suppression of emotions and the expression of emotion at the other end (Hunter, 2004, 2009). Staff shortages, time pressures and the rapid turnover of clients may contribute to feelings of emotional conflict and dissonance when the realities of the workplace contrast with the occupational and professional ideals and values of care providers (Hunter, 2004, 2010).

Other studies have shown how these external pressures can create emotional discord as the emphasis is on the efficient processing of tasks rather than engaging in the provision of personalised care underpinned by meaningful relationships, a source of frustration for both mothers and midwives (Edwards, 2010). Nurses also are often required to adapt their external exterior to accommodate their environment and minimise their personal feelings (Kirk, 2021). Recent survey findings have highlighted how both nurses and midwives suffer high levels of stress and burn-out within their workplace (NHS Survey, 2018, 2019), which may contribute to their decisions to leave the profession (Aiken et al., 2012; NHS Survey, 2018; Sermeus et al., 2011).

It is vital, therefore, that you pay careful attention to managing your emotions at work and develop strategies that might support you so that you can support clients and patients and prevent undue stress and burnout in yourself. Healthcare workers need to learn to adapt quickly within the practice setting as they respond to meet the needs of contrasting patient groups. Hiding personal distress and sadness can be a careful balancing act.

━━━━━━━━━━━ **ACTIVITY 5.1** ━━━━━━━━━━━

Reflection

Can you think of a situation when you had to hide your emotions?

Describe this event. What actions did you take to hide your feelings? Who else was involved and what did they do and say? How did this make you feel?

What did you do and how did you feel after the event?

Developing self-awareness

It is important to be aware of your emotions and the possible conflict that might occur between your own feelings and the organisational requirements of the workplace. Learning to negotiate the culture of your workplace and the associated emotions experienced within it takes time and patience. Organisational culture refers to the shared assumptions, values and beliefs which determine how people behave in organisations and encompasses all the unwritten rules and expectations of the workplace that as a student you may be unfamiliar with.

It is important to recognise that working with other people can be challenging and demanding. This requires that you treat yourself with compassion during these times and not feel despondent or demoralised if you have a negative emotional experience within practice. Remember that to be able to care compassionately for those using healthcare systems it is important that we first extend compassion to ourselves. Michael West and colleagues have examined the culture of the NHS workplace with emphasis on ensuring that we establish nurturing and compassionate care cultures for staff (West et al., 2017, 2019). Through their work they have identified three core elements required to create a compassionate and nurturing environment for health professionals and improve emotional wellbeing and resilience.

Core elements required to sustain emotional wellbeing within the workplace

Autonomy - Having a sense of control over your working environment
Belonging - Feeling valued and part of the team
Contribution - Having access to sufficient training to enable you to feel as though you are contributing to the workplace (West et al., 2019).

These elements will be discussed later in this chapter when we explore strategies for managing your emotions in more depth. As students you will learn to negotiate the path between acknowledging and reflecting upon your emotions within practice without being overwhelmed by them to enable you to practice compassionate awareness and empathy for those in your care. The well-known author Maya Angelou once said, *'I've learned that people will forget what you said, people will forget what you did, but people will never forget how you made them feel'*. These words may resonate with you and describe the powerful effect that the behaviours we encounter and our interactions with others may have on our emotions. It is well worth keeping these words in mind during your interactions with colleagues, patients and the wider public as you progress throughout your career in healthcare.

Understanding emotions in practice is essential for health and social care professionals. Emotions can be described as strong feelings derived from one's circumstances, mood or relationships with others (Oxford English Dictionary, ND). These can be in response to significant internal and external events, as well as in response to our relationships with others. They will be shaped and influenced by our unique previous experiences and personalities.

As a student, you may experience a variety of emotions when you first start your clinical placement, some of these may be positive, others might feel more negative. You may be excited that you are finally going to embark on the practical aspects of you chosen career. You may feel happy, fulfilled and valued, looking forward with anticipation to working with people or be feeling some anxiety (Figure 5.1).

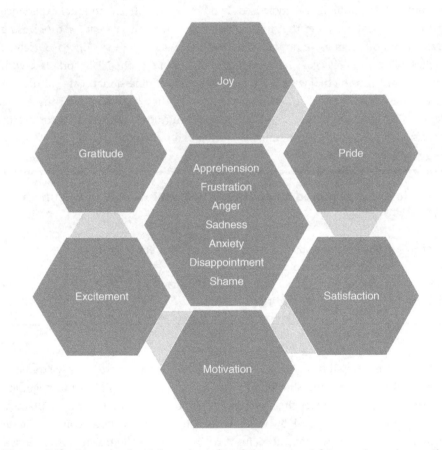

Figure 5.1 An example of the range of emotions you might experience in practice

You will have entered your profession with a variety of experiences which will influence your perception of yourself, of others and of practice. Case Study 5.1 outlines an example of how Emma's past experience might influence her emotional responses to care. Reflect upon this example as suggested below and complete.

Case study 5.1

Emma

Emma is a Year 1 student midwife. She gave birth to her son James two years ago and struggled to breastfeed. Emma remembers feeling unsupported and losing confidence in her ability to breastfeed. Emma also remembers feeling very disappointed and guilty that she was unable to continue to breastfeed. During her first day in practice, Emma was working in the community supporting new mothers with breastfeeding.

ACTIVITY 5.2

Critical Thinking and Reflection

Read and reflect upon Emma's situation. How do you think Emma might feel in this instance?

Consider how her earlier experiences with breastfeeding might affect Emma's approach to care when supporting new mothers within the community.

Now consider you own personal experiences.

How might these influence your approach to practice. It may be that you are a school leaver or have many years' experiences in your own field. Each person brings something personal and unique from their own background and experiences.

Write some notes on what experiences have led you to decide on your chosen career. These may include your personal experiences of healthcare and any positive and negative experiences of care that you may have experienced.

How might these experiences influence your approach to others within your chosen profession?

We recommend you record this reflection within your professional journal to facilitate your professional development.

Respecting and Responding to Your Own Emotions

Recognise and accept that you will have an emotional response to the situations you find yourself in within the healthcare arena. This is normal as certain situations may trigger memories and responses to feelings you have experienced in the past within your own personal life story. It is important that you learn to reflect upon these emotional responses with patience and kindness towards yourselves knowing that you will develop the skills to be able to respond responsively and compassionately over time. Remember to remain positive and apply your attention to your interactions, reflecting on any emotions or responses that are evoked.

━━━━━━━━━━ **SCENARIO 5.1** ━━━━━━━━━━

It is 2 weeks before your first day in practice. You have not worked within a healthcare setting before and therefore you are unfamiliar with the environment. You are feeling slightly anxious. When you rang for your shift rota, the nurse said she was too busy to give it to you and you don't know who you are working with or your shift pattern. You don't want to phone back in case you are perceived as being a nuisance.

During your first day, you are late because you could not find any parking. Once handover is finished the emergency bell rings and you are unsure about what you should do. Your practice supervisor runs off to help with the emergency and you don't know if you should follow him as well. A doctor runs by and asks you to bring a drip stand to room 4 and you are not sure where to find this and do not know where room 4 is. You don't want to ask for fear of looking silly.

There are lots of staff members on the ward, but you are not sure of their names or roles. Your practice supervisor introduced himself at the beginning of the shift, but you now can't remember his name and don't know where he is. The phone keeps ringing, and you are anxious about whether you should answer it. You have not had a break since 7 am and it is now 11 am and you are hungry as you did not have time for breakfast before the start of the shift. Your practice supervisor finds you at last and asks you to help him with the drug round.

━━━━━━━━━━ **ACTIVITY 5.3** ━━━━━━━━━━

Critical Thinking

Read the second scenario presented.

Consider what emotions you might experience in this situation.

What do you think might help you manage any difficult feelings you might experience?

You may have listed in your answer feelings of anxiety, fear and shame. Some of these are a very normal response to a new and challenging situation. Other people may also be experiencing anxiety around you during this time. Anxiety is a common response to unfamiliar situations which may manifest in different ways. Various responses to anxiety may be physical and behavioural. Symptoms might include increased heart rate, sweating, lack of concentration and impaired cognitive function. People may withdraw or demonstrate inconsiderate behaviours that lack sensitivity.

Taking responsibility to advocate for yourself is an important skill. Consider who you need to ask to obtain the shift rota and do not be afraid to try again. Be proactive in taking steps to establish and maintain a positive working relationship with your practice supervisor (Elcock, 2020) and clarify any uncertainty in names, roles and responsibilities as early as possible. Identify the support that is available to you including peer support and other students who are in a similar position. Remember to ask about orientation to the new environment and have a notebook and pen with you to take notes if needed.

Advocating for yourself can be difficult within a busy environment. It may be that your supervisor has forgotten to allocate a break and speaking out may feel inappropriate when you can see that those around you are busy. Adjusting to work patterns can be stressful and cause tiredness; so it is important to ensure adequate sleep or rest before a shift.

There may be some situations in practice that you had not expected, you may also come across other people who are distressed, stressed and anxious, and in some situations you might face issues of death and bereavement. All these can take their emotional toll on you and learning new skills can be very tiring. In all areas of practice, you might encounter bereavement and encounter clients who have been bereaved. An example from practice is provided in Scenario 5.2 presented below.

SCENARIO 5.2

You are a third-year student nurse who has been looking after Ethel an 84-year-old lady suffering with pneumonia for the past 6 weeks who had responded positively to treatment and discharged home. You felt delighted about this at the time as you had developed a good relationship with Ethel and her family, and she always asked you about your studies and your family. Following your theory block you return to practice to find that Ethel has returned to the ward and her condition has deteriorated significantly. Ethel has caught an infection and is being treated with antibiotics. You are shocked to see Ethel who does not recognise you, looks very different and appears to be losing consciousness. You are reminded of your own grandmother who recently passed away. The charge nurse asks you to urgently contact Ethel's daughter as he is concerned that Ethel does not have much longer to live.

ACTIVITY 5.4

Critical Thinking

Read the scenario and undertake:

How might you feel about this situation?

What emotions are triggered by Ethel's case and how might you react?

Bereavement can be apparent in different areas of healthcare work, whether as a result of a patients' condition or the experiences of relatives or staff members. It can bring up difficult feelings when someone dies. Feeling sad may be a normal response but you may find it particularly difficult because of your own experiences. You may over identify with a client because they remind you of a previous experience and it may be difficult to distinguish your own from others emotions. It may be that there are some unresolved issues that you bring to your role as a student healthcare practitioner, and this may be at an unconscious level what drew you to the work within healthcare. While this may result in you being more empathetic, it may also trigger your own distress in an unhelpful way. It is important that you develop self-awareness around this.

As health professionals, we are trained to fix things for others to make them better, but in some situations, this may not be possible; however, it is important to remember our presence can be a huge help. For example, being able to listen to someone's experiences without judgement or feeling as though you can make it better is an important skill to learn which may provide opportunity for the bereaved person to feel that their experience is both acknowledged and validated.

Poor Practice: Interprofessional Conflict and Responding to Others

Achieving a work life balance can present challenges within practice. There may be situations within your personal life that conflict with the requirements of your professional practice. An example might include when your child-minder is unwell, and you need to leave the ward to provide childcare or you are the main caregiver for a sick relative. There may also be situations when you are unable to attend special events because of your shift rota. These are some of the examples where you might experience conflict. It is important to think through these issues and how best they can be managed. It is important to be honest with yourself and ensure that you are aware of and take care to ensure that you uphold the professional values set out for your profession, for example, the Code (NMC, 2015, updated 2018).

Getting used to a new work culture with its unwritten rules and rituals can be challenging. Working with others can sometimes involve areas of conflict and you may be unsure about your role when dealing with hierarchy and speaking out. Entering a healthcare profession often involves adjusting to a different hierarchy and culture. This may take some time to adjust to and for you to feel valued as a student. Shame may result in a diminishing of your sense of self and lead to feelings of inadequacy or failure and a loss of healthy pride and sense of achievement. It may also result in withdrawal, submission or blaming self or others.

As well as recognising these symptoms in yourself, it is important to be aware of how emotions may affect the behaviour of those around us. It is important to separate your own feelings from those of others and consider the causes of other people's behaviours. Taking the opportunity to pay attention to and understand the reasons for other people's behaviour helps us develop compassion in our response and attitudes to them and is helpful in building interpersonal relationships with both staff members and clients (West & Chowler, 2017). You may experience the emotions of others such as anger which might feel as though they are being directed at you. However, it is important to bear in mind that there may come from a place of personal distress in the other and not as a direct attack on you.

Communication is fundamental in all aspects of healthcare. Individuals communicate in a variety of ways both verbally and non-verbally and this may not always be what you expect. It is important to be aware of your own body language and that of others as we all send signals to others about how we are feeling. When you are talking to someone notice what happens to your body and that of the other person. Notice how changing your body language might change how you feel and influence the response of the other person. There may be times during your practice that you might feel uncomfortable, for example, if you observe poor communication or unprofessional behaviour.

It is important as a professional that you endeavour to uphold the professional values outlined within the NHS Constitution and your professional code of conduct. Practicing kindness, compassion and civility within all our interactions is crucial to ensuring that we practice within a culture of compassion and provide high quality care. Should you witness unprofessional behaviour you should escalate this to your practice supervisor, assessor or lecturer so that steps can be taken to minimise this. Working together to ensure healthcare professionals treat each other and those within their care with compassion and civility is an important part of national strategy and essential within healthcare practice. The Civility Saves Lives website shown in the resources section provides more information about how critical it is to embed these values and behaviours within practice. Consider also the reflective activity outlined below to help foster your emotional awareness.

▬▬▬ ACTIVITY 5.5 ▬▬▬

Reflective Awareness

Think of a time where you have felt really stressed.

How did you respond?

What behaviours did you show?

These are red flag symptoms that you may exhibit which warn you that you may be feeling stressed and under pressure.

If you find yourself feeling overwhelmed with strong emotions. It is important to reflect and consider what might be the trigger for these emotions from your personal experiences.

Strategies to support your emotional wellbeing

Within this section we will consider various strategies that can be used to support your emotional health and wellbeing. Remember to not adopt a one size fits all approach as you may find some strategies are more beneficial than others. The key to managing your own emotions is to be aware of what you are feeling and how you respond to situations that might be more difficult. It is important to give yourself space to think about your own needs.

- Self-care. Remember that it is important to look after yourself. Being proactive and ensuring that you take steps to eat well, hydrate, exercise, ensure sufficient sleep and develop social support networks. One of the strategies that has been found to be helpful is a mindfulness practice. Mindfulness is a useful tool in all walks of life – it involves purposefully paying attention to the present moment in a non-judgmental way. It consists of observing what is happening moment by moment in one's internal (thoughts, motives, emotions, bodily sensations) and external world without judging it (Pena -sarrionadia et al., 2015).
- Journal writing and the practice of gratitude – sometimes it is helpful to write your thoughts and feelings down. If it is helpful, you may find using a reflective model beneficial to help guide you. Taking time to be appreciative and reflect upon what you have is important. Pay attention to the things that bring joy to your life. These may include your family, friends, garden, sunshine, nature, hobbies and interests. Reflecting can also help us develop our own personal knowledge of ourselves and responses to others.
- Do not underestimate the contribution that you can make to your team and your peers. Your voice matters. Planning your resources and being aware of the options available to you as well as being organised will help you feel as though you have control over your work-life balance. This will enhance your sense of autonomy, belonging and overall sense of contribution. These are all elements that have been shown to support resilience and promote your wellbeing.
- Clinical Supervision and Peer Support – your group may be going through the same emotional experiences as you and can be a useful source of support. It is important that you support each other and schedule time to check in with each other. In practice you will find support from your link teacher, personal tutor, supervisor, professional nurse or midwife advocate and other practitioners that you work with. Learning how to navigate the various support avenues available to you is important. You may access different support mechanisms for different issues. Your university wellbeing team, student union and student advisors will also be able to sign post you to appropriate support. Student buddies from other year groups can also be a helpful source of support.
- What do when things become difficult – Remember to access the support services available at your university as well as the 24-hour support that may be available. Examples of ways you could access support are included in the box below.

Examples of support

i. Your child is unwell, and you are becoming increasingly anxious about completing your course work in time: Speak to your personal tutor and student support team at your university or place of study to see what support is available to you to help you manage your deadlines.

ii. You go home from a shift in tears and are having trouble sleeping because of an experience at work: Reach out to your peers and family for support if available. You may need to speak with your GP or access the counselling services that may be available at your place of work or study.

iii. You think your mental health is deteriorating. You are increasingly anxious and find it difficult to concentrate. Your partner is unsupportive: Access your GP and the wellbeing team at your place of study without delay. Let your personal tutor know and inform your practice supervisor, practice assessor within practice that you are experiencing difficulties and require support. Remember to also access the 24-hour support that is available, for example, via the Samaritans or crisis line.

Chapter Summary

This chapter has focused on the nature of caring and the emotions that you may experience as a student embarking upon a career within healthcare. As a healthcare professional you will find yourself in many different privileged positions where you have opportunities to make a positive impact on the lives of others. You will bring a wealth of individual experience into the profession with you which may shape your responses and the emotions that are evoked through certain situations. Throughout your course you will develop your communication and interpersonal skills as you learn to combine the elements of professionalism with the emotional elements of care. This chapter has emphasised the importance of paying attention to and developing your emotional awareness at the start of your career in healthcare. Through doing so it will help enable you to positively manage your emotions and develop the human elements of authentic care and compassion while ensuring you protect against burn out and compassion fatigue.

6

Becoming Emotionally Intelligent

Raquel Marta and
Annette Chowthi-Williams

NMC Standards of Proficiency for Registered Nurses (NMC, 2018)
Professional Standards Social Work England (2019)
Standards of Proficiency (HCPC, 2018)

Nursing & Midwifery Council

This chapter will address the following platforms and proficiencies:

1 Being an accountable professional
2 Promoting health and preventing ill health
5 Leading and managing nursing care and working in teams
6 Improving safety and quality of care
7 Coordinating care

Social work England

This chapter will address the following standards:

Standard 1: Promote the rights, strengths and wellbeing of people, families and
communities
Standard 3: Be accountable for the quality of my practice and the decisions I make
Standard 4: Maintain my continuing professional development
Standard 5: Act safely and with professional integrity

Health and Care Professional Council

This chapter will address the following proficiencies:

1   Be able to practise safely and effectively within their scope of practice
3   Be able to maintain fitness to practise
5   Be aware of the impact of culture, equality and diversity on practice
8   Be able to communicate effectively
9   Be able to work appropriately with others
11 Be able to reflect on and review practice
12 Be able to assure the quality of their practice

Chapter aims

After reading this chapter, you will be able to:

- Understand the concept of emotional intelligence in social and healthcare.
- Develop self-awareness strategies to manage your own emotions and others.
- Distinguish the many factors that might impact our emotions in the workplace.
- Acquire knowledge and practical solutions on building positive personal and
  professional relationships in the workplace.
- Illustrate how to manage your own emotions in the workplace through effective
  leadership.

Introduction

In this chapter, we consider the question of what is emotional intelligence (EI) and
explore some basics of EI to help you understand the major characteristics and gain
insight into how to nurture the development of emotional self-strategies. With
leadership being a core skill for health and social care professionals, how we come to
incorporate skills and abilities derived from EI into leadership in professional
practice will also be discussed and explored. An essential foundation for a successful

professional performance is the awareness of what emotions are; how they can be managed, developed, and used in ourselves and in others. Emotions are part of our daily life and, as social and healthcare students and future leaders, it is essential that you nurture EI both in your professional and personal life. We provide strategies and resources to help you become emotionally intelligent.

What is Emotional Intelligence?

EI is ubiquitously in our daily lives and is rapidly becoming primordial for health and social care professions, where the relational essence is at its core. The human emotional arena is complex as emotions vibrate in our minds, radiate in our bodies, resonate through ourselves and are present in our personal and professional inter-action with others.

The study of EI is relatively recent. Complex and without consensus on its definition (Kotsou et al., 2019). Salovey and Mayer were the first authors to describe EI as the 'ability to monitor one's own and others' feelings and emotions, to discriminate among them and use this information to guide one's thinking and actions' (Salovey & Mayer, 1990, p. 267). The authors suggested that our various ways of engagement with emotions allows us to boost thinking, judgement, and inner and inter-behaviour, and since then, various scholars and EI models have emerged, always underlying the link between emotion and cognition (Mayer et al., 1999; Salovey & Mayer, 1990). In underlying such correlation, Daniel Goleman (1995) discussed EI as an intermingling of cognitive intelligence, emotion associated skills and personality attributes that, all together, allow us to contribute to one's personal and professional success in an adaptative and balanced manner.

The diagram (Figure 6.1) illustrates the major integrated abilities–traits needed to nurture EI as suggested by Goleman (1995, 1998; Serrat, 2017):

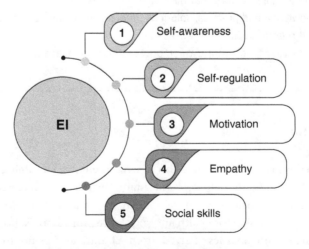

Figure 6.1 Five major traits of emotional intelligence

The nature of these traits is as following:

1. Self-awareness corresponds to an ongoing process of awareness of what is it that you feel, why you feel it and how you address such an emotional state. It is an inner invitation to know yourself, both in your strengths and weaknesses, and to nurture your sense of self-worth and self-confidence.

2. Self-regulation involves attributes of a regulatory nature, such as self-control, transparency, adaptability, initiative and optimism. It allows you to control emotional impulsiveness and to face and overcome emotional stressful situations.

3. Motivation is a source of optimism and persistence that emphasises the ability to be emotionally controlled – delaying reward and mastering impulsiveness – to achieve your goals. The conviction is that one dominates the events of one's life and is capable of overcoming challenges. Developing this skill will allow you to take risks and face challenges in working towards achieving your goals.

4. Empathy, the ability to recognise what others feel, plays a key role in a wide range of areas of life. It emerges from the emotional self-consciousness, as only by being able to recognise our own emotions, will we be able to recognise those of others. Empathic people are more sensitive to verbal and non-verbal clues and signals – including micro expressions – that indicate other feelings or needs. It is the technical term for describing the ability to 'put yourself in another person's shoes', considering the diverse backgrounds and life experiences, intuitively feeling what they are feeling, being able to consider their perspective, and nurturing the connection and the relationship.

5. Social skills are defined by our ability to understand or influence others' emotions. They enable us to manage emotions within relationships, thus providing us with the necessary accuracy in reading social situations. As you will see later in the chapter, it is an important leadership competence, as it encompasses the ability to persuade, lead, negotiate and promote cooperation.

━━━━━━━━━ **ACTIVITY 6.1** ━━━━━━━━━

Knowledge

Click on the link below and choose one of the different streaming platforms to listen to the Super Soul podcast with Daniel Goldman (2018):

https://www.oprah.com/own-podcasts/daniel-goleman-emotional-intelligence-101

Engage yourself with the conversation and identify three questions to discuss with your peers.

Knowing one's own emotions

As you have learnt in Chapter 4, emotions need to be understood as the intertwining of mind and brain, so knowing our own emotions is also associated with the ability to think, and this includes the aptitude to differentiate between emotional states and reflect upon the sources of these feelings. This emotional self-conscience implies the ability to identify, to reflect and to name emotions (Codier, 2020; Maye, 1990), allowing us to find what Ekman calls 'insight in awareness'. When you are capable of reflecting and verbalising what you feel, your emotional development takes on a whole new dimension: by being able to label your feelings, you manage to distance yourself from them, and you are capable of thinking about them. As Ekman (2003) suggests, the thinker behind the basic emotion theory underpins how emotions allow the analysis of information from the sensory organs which alert us to any situation that might happen (real, illusory or re-lived). In this sense, emotions allow us to act quickly, working as shortcuts that activate the body's functions for allowing an effective response that proves to be vital for human needs, adjustments or even survival. Emotions have distinct modes of expression: they vary from person to person, and they vary on intensity, and on cultural and contextual appropriateness (Ekman, 1984, 1999). The breadth of emotions can be, therefore, broadly surprising and, consequently, choosing the right word to name it is a difficult task, but you can start by expanding your emotional language.

In Figure 6.2, you will find a short list of emotion vocabularies. For the purpose of this chapter and table, we are considering categorisations of emotions in accordance with the basic emotion theory as developed by Ekman (1992, 1999).

Anger Grumpy	Sadness Lonely	Fear Worried	Disgust Dislike	Embarrassment Isolated	Enjoyment Happiness
Frustrated	Heartbroken	Doubtful	Revulsion	Self-cosncieous	Love
Annoyed	Gloomy	Nervous	Loathing	Lonely	Relief
Defensive	Disappointed	Anxious	Disapproving	Inferior	Contentment
Spiteful	Hopeless	Terrified	Offended	Guilty	Amusement
Disgusted	Grieved	Panicked	Horrified	Ashamed	Joy
Offended	Unhappy	Horrified	Uncomfortable	Repugnant	Pride
Irritated	Lost	Desperate	Nauseated	Pathetic	Excitement
Impatient	Troubled	Confused	Disturbed	Confused	Peace
Mad	Resigned	Stressed	Withdrawal		Satisfaction
Vengeful	Miserable	Worried	Aversion		Compassion

Figure 6.2 Brief list of emotions

It is equally important to understand that, often, there are emotions that we struggle to explain. This animated video about *12 Emotions You Might Feel But Can't Explain* can help you comprehend some of these emotions https://www.youtube.com/watch?v=bny9YViO15o&t=119s.

━━━━━━━━ **ACTIVITY 6.2** ━━━━━━━━

Reflection and Practice

Understanding yourself, knowing your own emotions, is an ongoing process that requires becoming self-aware of weakness, blurred behaviour, strengths and positive traits that impact your wellbeing, your inter-relational behaviour, your emphatic skills and your professional performance. In Figure 6.3, you find a non-exhaustive list of traits. Take time to reflect, think about your daily behaviour or situations that you have experienced and identify six traits that correspond to your strengths and six that you think would be beneficial to expand. Justify the reasons for your choices. Remember that experiences throughout life shape the way our mind and, consequently, our emotions work, so the traits are not static, they are continually developing.

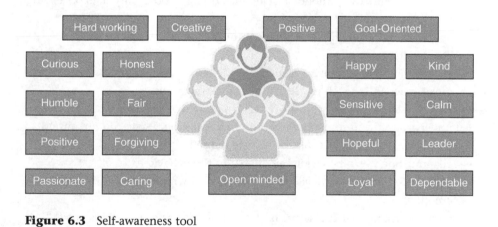

Figure 6.3 Self-awareness tool

Recognising emotions in others

Emotions, as described by Damasio (2018), consists of subjectively experienced psychic and physical extensions that are triggered by a stimulus. This means that emotions are a natural way of evaluating the environment that activates us and reacts adaptively. On the same note, Juckel et al. (2019) highlight that the process of observing emotions is not done in isolation, it is dependent on the context, of both the internal and external environment. The identification and recognition of the facial expression of emotion involves, then, not only the information that we are looking at in the other person's face but also as the foreknowledge we have of the emotion that we are perceiving in the other. We all can identify facial expressions like sadness, joy, disappointment, fear and so on but feelings – and the emotions that they trigger – always cover some mode of language, sometimes hidden or inhibited (Codier, 2020; Damasio, 2018; Juckel et al., 2019; Serrat, 2017).

Although the tradition of emotions has been understood in terms of the bodily sensations, the reading or decoding of emotional expression through the body is not always possible *per se*. Think about the members of a jazz band, how they synchronise when improvising to achieve one melody only. Face-to-face interaction in social and healthcare requires the same type of ability: the one that allows us to perceive the actions of others – such as silence, passivity, sonority, noise – interpret them, and react accordingly, with the aim of constructing mutually congruent interactional moments, share emotional meanings and develop joint answers. To achieve such a goal, and having presented that the differentiation of emotions in others cannot occur without understanding and recognising your own – a core component of empathy – it is important to develop emotional competence towards the others, which requires:

- perceiving one's own emotional state, including the possibility of experiencing multiple emotions
- appreciating the emotions of others, through non-verbal expressions and/or behaviours
- using emotional vocabulary adequate to the other's culture and be emotionally sensitive when interacting with vulnerable populations
- engaging empathically with the others' emotional experience
- understanding and recognising that internal emotional states do not always correspond to the expressions being externalised
- adapting one's own behaviour emotional to the behaviours of others
- using self-regulatory strategies to adaptively deal with adverse or disruptive emotions
- comprehending that the nature of the interactions or relationships depend on the degree of emotional genuineness in their manifestation and the degree of reciprocity in the relationship.

━━━━━━━━━ **ACTIVITY 6.3** ━━━━━━━━━

Reflection and Practice

Are you wondering how emotionally intelligent are you? This activity is for you: click on the link below to perform a self-assessment of how emotionally intelligent you are. You are required to read each statement and answer accordingly.

https://www.mindtools.com/pages/article/ei-quiz.htm

As you finish, click on 'Calculate my total' and reflect on your results. Try to do it every 3 months and take note and reflect on the variations.

Leading and Managing One's Own Emotions

Self-leadership

In healthcare, leadership has become an essential criterion for all professionals and as future practitioners you will need to not only lead yourself but will become leaders and thus will need to develop a range of skills and competencies to both self-lead and effectively lead others. Every aspect of healthcare requires leadership, and many professional statutory bodies have set out the importance of self-leadership and leading others and some have outlined leadership and self-leadership as competencies.

What is self-leadership and why is self-leadership so important for you as practitioners in health and social care?

Self- leadership is about:

- each of us knowing who we are
  - what we are capable of doing and achieving
  - what our aspirations are
  - being able to affect how we relate to others
  - how we manage our emotions and behaviour as we journey through our personal and professional life (Bryant & Kazan, 2012).

The notion of self-leadership was originally defined as a 'comprehensive self-influencing perspective that concerns leading oneself' (Manz, 1983, p. 594). It is evident from these definitions, that self-leaders deliberately guide how they think, feel and act in relation to their plans; in other words they are self-influencers. The individuals thus seek to lead themselves.

https://www.youtube.com/watch?v=4MOsteGgo0o

━━━━━ ACTIVITY 6.4 ━━━━━

Critical Thinking

Using this definition, consider the activity below. Give yourself time to answer the questions.

Think about you and answer these questions

Who are you?

What are you capable of doing?

What are your aspirations?

Can you think of a situation when your communication skills, emotions and behaviour enabled you to influence someone towards a different decision?

While undertaking the activities you may have found it a challenge answering the question of who you are, what you can do and your future plans or you may have found it easy. Knowing yourself could help you feel more at ease caring for others as well as working in a team where communication is at the heart of every aspect of your work as well as having to manage your emotions at all levels in the workplace. You may well encounter conflict with colleagues, the team or having to deal with stressful situations regarding patients, service users and clients. Thus, knowing yourself and your abilities will aid you in addressing future challenges. It means that if you are able to identify areas of yourself that needs developing, you can take up opportunities in your organisation to develop your skills and competence.

In reviewing the literature for their studies van Dorssen et al. (2021) and Kayal and Dulger (2019) discussed three self-leadership strategies that are used by people who are self-influencers. These are behavioural-focused, constructive thought pattern and natural reward strategies. Behavioural-focused strategies they suggest involves the individual trying to direct how they behave and does so through noticing how they are behaving and shaping their behaviour either through self-punishment or self-rewards. They may take actions such as setting themselves targets, listing activities to achieve and may have motivational visuals around their environment to keep them motivated. On the other hand, if they have not achieved their goals, they may deny themselves something that was pleasurable.

In regard to constructive thought pattern strategies, the individual focuses on positive solutions, blocking out negative thoughts and do not spend their time dwelling on the past. Their actions might involve self-talk, they might imagine their role in achieving their goal successfully and often spend time thinking carefully about things. The final strategy is natural reward strategy which uses both the behavioural and cognitive aspects. This strategy involves the individual viewing the activities they have to do in a positive way and mentally putting efforts into making these activities gratifying and rewarding. They tend to concentrate on the part of the job that gives them satisfaction.

These researchers have pointed to studies on self-leadership and the outcomes. This kind of leadership is linked with positive outcome for people working in healthcare organisations. People who are self-leaders tend to be engaged in their job and are more satisfied with the work they do, are more successful in terms of promotion as well have beneficial health outcomes. In their research, Kayal and Dulger (2019) found that self-leadership skills were a key part of attaining the organisation's targets. They highlighted aspects of patient safety, efficiency and productivity. van Dorssen et al. (2021) study indicate a similar outcome. However, these studies were exploring the impact of self-leadership training. With such benefits to self-leadership, it might be the case that individuals may well want to explore undertaking training and development programmes to improve their self-leadership abilities.

Leadership: Leading others

Having gained a sense of what self-leadership means and your own self-leadership status, leading others may become less of a challenge. Leading is another essential skill needed as a practitioner. In health and social care leadership can take the form of leading others, leading a team, a meeting, a case conference, a project, leading major change or leading on professional issues.

With such responsibilities of leading, people are more likely to respond if leaders lead with EI. There are many researchers, academics and writers who believe that leading with EI makes for effective leadership and certain styles of leadership may lead with EI. Whatever style of leadership is used, leading with EI will achieve better results. However, it is not easy to manage our emotions effectively especially when faced with challenging people or situations. In this chapter and in Chapters 4 and 5 we have given you tips on managing your emotions.

The question of whether leaders are born or made is still in debate. However, there are many different styles of leadership that can be adopted by practitioners. This will require individuals to decide which one is appropriate and that will depend on the individual's judgement of the situation, event, the size and scope of teams, the setting, goals and targets of the organisations as well as many other factors.

Northouse (2013) defines leadership as a 'process whereby an individual influences a group of individuals to achieve a common goal'.

━━━━━━━━━━ **ACTIVITY 6.5** ━━━━━━━━━━

Critical Thinking

Think about kind of leader you are?

How did you become the kind of leader you are presently?

What are your thoughts about leader being born or made?

Democratic leaders tend to involve and consult with people, in so doing the opportunity is there to acknowledge others' emotions, address these and manage your own emotions as you respond to people's views and opinions. Whereas autocratic leaders tend to give orders to people and there are dangers in this approach of not acknowledging your own emotions or other people's emotions. Such situations might create negative emotional responses and such individuals may find that their instructions are not carried out. However, there are times that this style of leadership is needed. For example, in an emergency situation and in such situations, the team may well accept this style of leadership and see it as necessary in such events.

There are other leadership styles as indicated earlier. There are situational leaders, transformational, compassionate leaders and leaders as 'enablers'. These styles of leadership offer practitioners new ways of leading and opens up the opportunity to lead in a variety of ways. Transformational leaders tend to see opportunities for innovation, to bring about change in procedures, processes, the way the organisation works, introducing new approaches on how practitioners might work. This style of leadership is ideal in bringing about change through innovation and improvement. This style of leadership tends to focus highly on people, relationships, and in healthcare, people are its greatest resources. It's about mutual inspiration and motivation, discussion and engagement. This leadership approach leads to improved performance and improved group satisfaction, compared to other forms of leadership (Choi et al., 2016) and improved wellbeing (Arnold, 2017). Within the health services, evidence points to this kind of leadership resulting in improved job satisfaction, a better practice environment and improved nurse retention (West et al., 2015).

You may find in practice you see opportunities for doing things differently. Innovation and improvement are now a key part of the future nurse's role and thus many of these styles of leadership are apt for leading service change. You can learn more about healthcare innovation, improvement and development and the different styles of leadership in *Successful Change Management in Health Care* (2022) by Annette Chowthi-Williams and Geraldine Davis.

West et al. (2017) suggest in healthcare compassionate leadership can be effective when bringing about change. However, compassionate leadership is not just needed for change but in every aspect of leading. People prefer compassion from their leaders. Leaders who show care, empathy and concern for those they are leading are more likely to motivate people than leaders who simply give orders and instructions, though there is a place for autocratic leadership such as in an emergency situation. As a leader you will encounter people with diverse opinions, values and beliefs, and leadership is about gaining consensus, so that the highest quality of care can be delivered for patients, service users and clients.

Jabbal (2017) believes leaders should be 'enablers'. This approach is about leaders acting in the capacity of a facilitator, an organiser or an initiator. It involves leaders finding the means to help their workforce achieve their goals. Such leaders would need to provide the relevant resources such as training and education, allocated time, finance, mentorship and other support to help practitioners to undertake their roles.

━━━━━━━━━ **ACTIVITY 6.6** ━━━━━━━━━

Critical Thinking

Think of a situation, group or a service you have led.

Think of a situation, a group or a service that your practice supervisor assessor has led.

What style of leadership did you use and was it effective or not? Give your reasons.

What style of leadership did your practice supervisor/assessor use and was it effective or not? Give your reasons.

━━━━━━━━━━━ **ACTIVITY 6.7** ━━━━━━━━━━━

Reflection

Case study 6.1: Alan

Alan had a tough day in the GP practice with many patients in the diabetic clinic needing more time to discuss their results and next steps to managing their health and wellbeing. The practice manager interrupted his clinic and ordered him to clear out the room and equipment he used earlier. He responded by informing her that patients were more important which then led to a longer conversation which left both of them feeling unsettled.

Examine the different styles of leadership above and think about the following:

What leadership approach was used and what approach might have been appropriate in this situation?

Which leadership styles do you think can lead in an emotionally intelligent way? Why?

───────────────────────────────────

The autocratic style of leadership by the practice manager seems to have upset them both. Alan had intended to complete tidying the consultation room. He was right to put his patients first. Had the practice manager used a compassionate style of leadership approach, perhaps the subsequent conversation might not have been negative. It is clear the practice manager could have used emotional intelligence through being aware of how Alan might be feeling having had a busy day and was still seeing patients. She could have equally managed her own feelings by being aware that she was getting inpatient that he had not cleared up the consulting room and perhaps used a strategy to manage any negative feelings. EI is viewed as an important aspect of an effective leader and there is support for the idea that training can improve EI (Goleman, 1995, 2006; Northouse, 2018).

This is an interesting idea and many organisations worldwide provide training for leaders in this area. The Francis Report (2013) enquiry into the failings of the Mid Staffordshire NHS Foundation Trust found poor leadership to be a critical factor.

Many health and social care curricula have leadership development as a core theme in their education and training programmes. The NHS has recognised the importance of effective leadership. The NHS Leadership Model has been developed and it is available for everyone to use. There are nine domains in the model. You can access it below and take the opportunity to assess your own leadership potential.

https://www.leadershipacademy.nhs.uk/resources/healthcare-leadership-model/

Chapter Summary

Emotions are part of our daily life, and as social and healthcare students and future leaders it is important that you are able to develop and maintain EI. Being aware of what emotions are; how they can be managed, developed and used personally and professionally has been a key part of this chapter. Whether you are self-leading or leading a team, being aware and managing your emotions is critical. We explored some basics of EI to help you understand the major characteristics and gain insight into how to nurture the development of emotional self-strategies. We further explored self-leadership the varying styles of leadership, all of which required us to manage our emotions effectively to get the best from those we are leading.

7

Building Resilience

Kate Nash and Annette Chowthi-Williams

NMC Standards of Proficiency for Registered Nurses (NMC, 2018)
Professional Standards Social Work England (2019)
Standards of Proficiency (HCPC, 2018)

Nursing & Midwifery Council

This chapter will address the following platforms and proficiencies:

1   Being an accountable professional
2   Promoting health and preventing ill health
3   Leading and managing nursing care and working in teams
6   Improving safety and quality of care

Social Work England

This chapter will address the following standards:

Standard 1: Promote the rights, strengths and wellbeing of people, families and communities
Standard 3: Be accountable for the quality of my practice and the decisions I make

Standard 4: Maintain my continuing professional development
Standard 5: Act safely and with professional integrity

Health and Care Professional Council

This chapter will address the following proficiencies:

1   Be able to practise safely and effectively within their scope of practice
3   Be able to maintain fitness to practise
9   Be able to work appropriately with others
11 Be able to reflect on and review practice
12 Be able to assure the quality of their practice
14 Be able to draw on appropriate knowledge and skills to inform practice

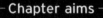

Chapter aims

Upon reading this chapter, you will be able to:

- Understand the concept of resilience in healthcare
- Gain knowledge and understanding about the various factors that might lead to stress and burnout
- Understand the strategies and practical solutions for dealing with stress in the workplace
- Gaining knowledge and insight on how to build resilience

Introduction

This chapter will examine the notion of resilience, its role and importance in enabling students to manage and deal with challenges, drawbacks and the unexpected. It will explore the research within the field of resilience and offer a step-by-step guide to developing resilience. Building upon the concepts of emotional intelligence this chapter will consider how practitioners can foster the skills for developing resilience as a strategy for managing challenges and enhancing emotional wellbeing within the workplace. The importance of building and maintaining resilience is stressed with available resources to support these aspects.

Understanding the Importance of Resilience

Resilience has not always been viewed as a significant feature in the life of healthcare professionals from the standpoint of the literature, healthcare practice, nursing practice and healthcare education. However, recently it has gained prominence in all arenas of health and social care. The Royal College of Nursing (RCN, 2017) recently held a debate on the subject, and it is now a feature of the pre-registration curricula (NMC, 2018). Healthcare and healthcare organisations have become complex, together with changes in patterns of disease, technological developments, changing government policies and the public expectation leading to a rise in demands upon health and social care professionals. This growing complexity has caused large numbers of professionals, especially nurses and midwives either leaving or contemplating leaving the profession, citing factors such as pay cuts, low morale, understaffing, poor work-life balance and poor working conditions.

Workplace stress is a major factor contributing to this situation, the emotional labour of the work of caring itself, the need to be compassionate, work overload and a shortage of resources. With the current situation of the COVID-19 pandemic, the need for healthcare students to understand resilience, its contributing factors and the need to build and to develop their resilience has gained even more importance now.

Health and social care professionals in their role are exposed daily to many physical, psychological and emotional events in the workplace that will require them to be resilient. Such situations may lead to anxiety, worry and increase in stress levels and may show themselves in how one feels and thinks physically, emotionally or psychologically. These feelings maybecome exacerbated at certain times. For example, while caring for individuals or groups, at team meetings, while working with others, being out visiting clients in the community and primary care where you may be witnessing the challenging social, emotional and environment conditions your clients live with daily. You may be dealing with clients who are seriously ill and are receiving palliative care. You may be involved in caring for people experiencing a mental health crisis or requiring urgent help and support. You may be addressing safeguarding issues relating to children, young people or adults.

The environment of health and social care is constantly changing. Since 2020, the COVID pandemic has brought about many new challenges in the health and social care setting. New ways of working have been emerging; patients, clients and service users demand has grown resulting in increased pressure on professionals to deliver instant services. Many practitioners are working longer hours, facing new challenges caring for the nation, not being able to take leave, even having to be away from their families and most crucially putting themselves and their families at risk. Many are having to deal with high levels of unexpected deaths of patients, of relatives, loved ones, their own mortality, illness themselves and yet are expected to continue in their role.

It is essential therefore that you as health and social care professionals have a good understanding of the notion of resilience and understand how you can develop and build your resilience. This is an integral component of becoming a health and social care professional in the 21st century and key to sustaining holistic wellbeing throughout your course of study and future practice.

━━━━━━━━ **ACTIVITY 7.1** ━━━━━━━━

Reflection – The Concept of Resilience

Can you think of someone who you believe to be resilient? It could be a public figure. Family member/friend/colleague?

Describe this individual

What factors contributed to this individual's resilience?

Some experts believe that we inherit resilience, while others think it is something that is built up as we go through varying experiences. According to Hone (2017) resilience should not be seen as a 'fixed trait', which some people possess, and others do not have. Resilience is something that is attainable and achievable for everyone. Becoming resilient then requires putting into action routine and regular practices. It means people have to be motivated, prepared to undertake the hard work to help them become resilient. While individual experts have sought to give their own definition of resilience, there are common features among writers and experts. Paul McKenna (2022) tells us that, it involves how we think. Therefore we need to adapt and adjust, become innovative and 'resourceful'.

The National Health Service (NHS) Leadership Academy (2022) suggests that being resilient is about people being able to 'bounce-back' from experiencing hardships whereby they are then able to adjust themselves, their feelings, thoughts, behaviour and continue to flourish. Webb (2020) defines the notion in a number of ways. It could be the progression of 'adapting' and 'recovering' as we experience events and situations. She further suggests that it could also be about people having the capacity to 'bend' as opposed to 'break' or people persisting, continuing and adapting when confronted by difficulties. It's worth noting that these writers use similar language to define the notion of resilience. A common theme is recovery after having experienced a change in whatever form that might take – a loss of loved one, break up of a relationship or failing your exam.

Being resilient then is about the individual being able to adapt in the face of serious challenges, having the ability to handle difficult situation in a positive manner, thinking innovatively and finding opportunities and solutions to current challenges. It is about having positive thoughts, feelings and behaviours and using these to help you through adverse events or situations. But what do these ideas mean for health and social care students? As future health professionals it means that you will need to adapt to a new learning environment, different work settings, working with a diverse range of professionals, the demands of caring for patients, clients and service users, stressful situations and conflicts. There will be constant change as you progress through your education and training. However, these are all normal challenges of joining one of the most rewarding professions. The key is to develop and maintain your resilience. Be resourceful and be innovative and inventive by looking for personal and professional solutions with others, look after your health, think positive, seek help from the many sources in your university and in your practice setting and be proactive. In the face of the change, these actions will enable you to cope and thrive in your professional and personal life.

================ ACTIVITY 7.2 ================

Reflection – Reflecting on Your Own Resilience

Thinking about yourself and your own resilience.

- Can you identify a time when you had to face a serious challenge?
- Describe this situation?
- Describe how to deal with this event, i.e. the actions/the activities you undertook to help yourself recover
- Do you feel that you are resilient or becoming more resilient?

An interesting question to ponder on is this. What then helps us to become resilient and what hinders our resilience in our personal and professional life. Figure 7.1 illustrates some factors within the context of health and social care that may promote resilience and Figure 7.2 illustrates the factors that might hinder resilience.

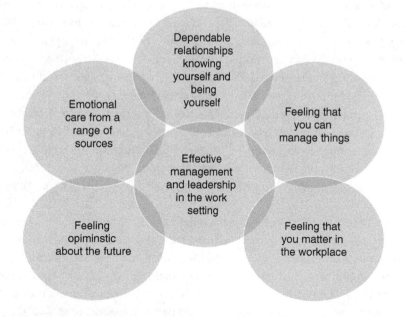

Figure 7.1 Factors that promote resilience

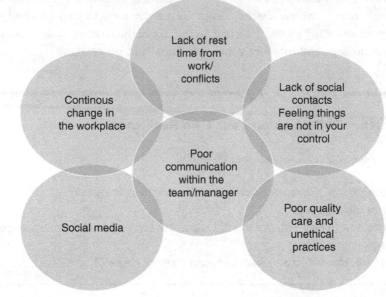

Figure 7.2   Factors that might hinder our ability to be resilient

Stress and Burnout Within Healthcare Professionals

The previous chapters have highlighted how the emotional work of caring can contribute to stress and burnout within health professionals. Stress can be defined as the adverse reaction that people may have to excessive pressures or other types of demand placed upon them (The Health and Safety Executive, 2017). Work-related stress is a key cause of ill health within the workplace and can contribute to severe physical and psychological conditions. Stress is known to be more prevalent in public service occupations, such as health and social care (NHS Employers, 2021). Within the NHS stress, anxiety and depression, along with other mental health conditions remain consistently the most reported reason for sickness absence, accounting for over 442,500 full time equivalent days lost and 28.6% of all sickness absence in September 2020 (NHS Digital, 2021). Overall, approximately 40% of all staff sickness absence in the entire NHS is due to work-related stress with an associated cost to the NHS of up to £400 million per year (Rimmer, 2018).

The global COVID pandemic has shone light on the importance of safeguarding the health and wellbeing of all healthcare workers and ensuring organisations have processes in place for doing this. While the notion of stress and burnout within healthcare is not new, it is anticipated that existing levels of work-related health problems are likely to rise further. This is partly due to the exceptional pressures that many practitioners are experiencing during the pandemic (Kinman et al., 2020; NHS

Confederation 2020) which are compounded further by a lack of resources and the chronic excessive workload that may be experienced in practice (Hunter et al., 2018; West et al., 2020). Understanding the basic core needs of NHS staff and health practitioners is vital to ensure that they are being met for the sake of staff wellbeing and the ability to provide compassionate, high-quality care as discussed within Chapter 5 (West et al., 2017).

Stress is something that everyone feels at times although it does affect people differently and can be experienced differently on an individual basis and manifest itself in a variety of ways. The experience of stress may be affected by factors such as age, experience, support factors, personal circumstances and health. While stress itself is not an illness, over time, if severe stress continues, it may lead to mental health conditions such as depression or anxiety and cause illness. Being alert and aware of early indicators of stress or *red flags* can help ensure that you plan intervention in a timely way enabling you to decompress and reduce stress before adverse effects occur. Burnout is described as a syndrome of emotional exhaustion and depersonalisation which occurs among workers who are involved in close human relationships often in response to chronic emotional strain and sometimes called compassion fatigue. It may manifest as a callous or unfeeling attitude towards clients and individuals suffering from burnout may hold negative self-perceptions of their achievements and undermine their personal accomplishments (Maslach & Jackson, 1981; Upton, 2018).

NHS and healthcare organisations have an important role to play in supporting their workforce and ensuring that strategies and processes are in place to help staff manage stress effectively. Many healthcare trusts have taken steps to invest in the health and wellbeing of staff and created wellbeing hubs and other initiatives to help staff manage what is often an inherently stressful and demanding role within healthcare. This is important as the emotional and psychological wellbeing of staff has a direct impact on the care of patients, professional relationships, staff retention and our ability to flourish and effectively meet the challenges faced within the workplace (National Workforce Skills Development Unit, NWSDU, 2019).

Work factors associated with stress and burnout

The causes of stress may be internal or external. Internal factors may be related to a person's characteristics and personality traits and are usually self-generated, while external factors are factors existing as stimuli outside of the individual. Work factors associated with stress and occupational burnout include a perceived loss of autonomy and job control, lack of teamwork, feeling unsafe, a perception of reduced support and organisational factors such as shift working, heavy workload, bullying, poor quality support and staff shortages (De Hert, 2020; Kirkham et al., 2006; Mollart et al., 2011). Chronic workplace stress has the potential to negatively influence both the health of employees and the wider organisation, and in the context of healthcare, it also may also negatively impact upon patient care and health outcomes.

Human factors encompass all those factors that can influence people and their behaviour. Acknowledged as an essential part of keeping people safe, the Clinical Human Factors Group (2013) define human factors as the science of understanding human performance within a given system. Within the context of our working lives, these are the environmental, organisational and individual characteristics which influence behaviour at work and can be a cause of significant stress and burnout.

Understanding how human factors can influence care is important as human factors are a significant contributor to adverse events within healthcare. All healthcare workers need to have a basic understanding of human factors principles within healthcare. As human beings we are fallible and our performance at work can be affected by our personal life experiences, external pressures and a lack of a robust support structures. We need to be alert to these factors and recognise that mistakes can be made regardless of our experience, intelligence, motivation, or vigilance. The SHEEP acronym developed by Rosenorn-Lanng (2014) is a useful way of categorising the range of human factors that we may encounter within the clinical environment. These are outlined within Table 7.1. While these human factors can both contribute to and cause stress and burnout, the experience or manifestation of stress itself is also a human factor that can negatively influence our performance.

Table 7.1 Categories of human factors adapted from the SHEEP acronym (Rosenorn-Lanng, 2014)

Systems	These are the systems and processes within your place of work which include standard operating procedures, workforce rotas, daily management of the clinical area and escalation processes. Taking time to familiarise yourself with guidelines and protocols may help to familiarise you with the operational management of the clinical area.
Human interactions	Non-technical skills like leadership, teamwork, workload management and communication play an important role in improving patient safety and are influential human factors that if suboptimal may contribute significantly to stress.
Environment	The environment can influence your performance and it is important to be alert to distractions such as noise, buzzers, lighting, trip hazards and heating. Ensure that you dress appropriately and have had opportunity for orientation to the clinical area at the start of your placement.

Table 7.1 Categories of human factors adapted from the SHEEP acronym (Rosenorn-anng, 2014) *(Continued)*

Equipment	Equipment should be clinically effective, safe and meet the needs of the people that will use it and be treated by it. Check that equipment is in working order, appropriate for the task at hand, recently calibrated and sufficient trained if its undertaken. Ward areas should have checklists that your mentor or supervisor will be able to talk you through.
Personal factors	Personal factors such as life events, bereavement, stress, fatigue, values, attitudes, emotions and pathology and physiology may all affect behaviours under pressure. Be sure to alert your mentor, supervisor or tutor so that you can be signposted to support and guidance to help you navigate these life events.

Taking preventative steps and action to manage stress may prevent further escalation from stress to distress and the consequent detrimental impact it may have upon your clinical practice, personal health and wellbeing. Developing self-awareness and taking time to notice both your own responses to stress as well as those triggers that might cause you to feel stress forms a crucial part of your toolkit for managing your stress levels. It is important also to be alert to signs of stress demonstrated by your peers and colleagues and encourage them to take action, particularly if they appear to be demonstrating signs that they are not coping. Initial indicators that may cause you to suspect that yourself or others are experiencing escalating stress levels are summarised within the box below.

Initial indicators of increasing stress levels (adapted from Health and Safety Executive (2021) and The Chartered Institute of Personnel and Development (CIPD))

- Reports of stress, sickness, non-attendance, and absence and withdrawal from work and social events, leaving early
- Changes in character, becoming withdrawn and feeling reluctant to engage, feelings of ambivalence, having difficulties prioritising and making decisions
- Difficulties with time management and persistent lateness
- Increased emotional reactions, for example, becoming aggressive or more tearful than usual, unusual sensitivity, bullying behaviour
- Deterioration in work performance, for example, skipping breaks, loss of motivation, commitment and confidence
- Increased alcohol or nicotine intake or other substance misuse, change in physical appearance, loss of interest, accidents at home or the workplace. Changes in demeanour, for example, agitation, sweating, appearing anxious

Increasing your stress awareness and taking steps to manage your stress.

━━━━━━━━━━━ **ACTIVITY 7.3** ━━━━━━━━━━━

Reflection – Responding to Pressure

Compile a list of the physical and emotional signs that you exhibit when under pressure. This will help you to recognise these signs as red flags that can alert you to your increasing stress levels. Following this consider your automatic response to stress and consider how you can take steps to proactively adopt positive measures that will enhance your health and wellbeing.

━━━━━━━━━━━ **ACTIVITY 7.4** ━━━━━━━━━━━

Reflection – Managing Stress Positively

- List some of the habits you engage in when feeling stressed?
- Consider whether these habits enhance or are detrimental to your overall health and wellbeing.
- What kind of small changes can you invest in to improve your health? (Better sleep, better nutrition, hydration, exercise)
- What strategies might you use in your day-to-day life to improve your physical health and psychological wellbeing?
- List one small change you can make right now.
- What impact do you think this might have on your wellbeing?

Managing Stress Within the Workplace

Professional bodies have emphasised the importance of healthy working environments and have called for organisations to create better work environments for their employees. The Healthy Workplace toolkit (RCN, 2021) defines a healthy workplace as one which offers fair pay and rewards and has high-quality employment practices and procedures which are inclusive, promote a good work-life balance, protect and promote employees' physical and psychological health, facilitate employee autonomy and control as well as providing equitable access to training and learning and development.

The impact of fatigue on practice has been highlighted as a significant human factor and is a key safety issue (RCN, 2022). Not having opportunity for sufficient rest and recuperation can be detrimental and a link between staff burnout and not taking adequate quality breaks has been found (Germaine et al., 2021). Issues such as lack of flexible working, long shifts and work pressures have also been highlighted (Kinman et al., 2020).

In practice, practitioners may work through their breaks within practice due to workload and reduced staffing. Staff may also feel under pressure to work through their breaks when busy due to feelings of guilt if their colleagues appear busy (Germaine et al., 2021). Ensuring you take regular rest breaks is important. The concept of resilience should not endorse a work culture where endurance is tested, and practitioners expected to toughen up and remain silent when working within challenging conditions (Crowther et al., 2016). Instead, practitioners should be encouraged to develop skills and strategies that enhance personal health and well-being and nurture emotional strength and awareness, a positive sense of self and connectivity and compassion towards others. This includes speaking out and esca-lating when working under pressurised conditions that may negatively affect your wellbeing and have a detrimental impact on patient safety.

Examples of good practice include a campaign to use HALT (textbox 2) as a trigger for clinical staff to take regular breaks. The anacronym stands for Hungry, Angry, Late and Tired (HALT) and helps to remind practitioners of factors that may negatively influence their performance and to promote a positive culture where members of staff are supported to ensure they have opportunity for sufficient rest and restoration (Ragau et al., 2018).

Don't forget Halt if you are:

H ungry
A ngry
L ate or
T ired

(adapted from Ragau et al., 2018)

It is important also to bear in mind that there may be occasions where because of the duty of care you owe your patients it may be unsafe to take a break in certain circumstances. Understanding accountability is an important part of your profes-sional training. As a qualified practitioner there is a requirement to promote profes-sionalism at all times and ensure that your acts and omissions do not compromise the safety of those in your care. It is important to speak out if you have concerns about working under unsustainable pressures meaning that you cannot take breaks during your working day (RCN, 2021). Such concerns can be escalated via the ward or area manager, your personal tutor or through your local professional representative. The RCN Workforce Standards (RCN, 2021) are intended to support a safe and effective nursing workforce and include guidance on workforce planning and rostering, as well as staff health, safety and wellbeing. A summary is provided in textbox 3.

Workforce Standards (Adapted from the RCN, 2022)

You are entitled to a minimum break of 20 minutes when your daily working time is more than 6 hours which should be uninterrupted, not at the start or the end of the day and away from the work station.

Regulations generally require that there should be a break of 11 consecutive hours between each 12-hour shift.

The RCN believe that no shift should be longer than 12 hours and that 12-hour shifts may not be appropriate for all nurses and need to be considered in the context of patient safety and the physical and psychological demands of shift work.

Developing Your Strategies Toolkit for Promoting Resilience

It is important when faced with challenges that we acknowledge and address these, not simply pushing these away. It is normal to feel anxiety and worries as you start your course. These may be about meeting new people, making friends, wondering about how you will cope in your new environment, whether you will cope with your studies and be able to care for patients and service users. Experiencing negative feelings may and will arise in our thoughts and behaviours. This is not abnormal but remaining calm and pulling on your strength and resources and being positive will help to deal with events. Whatever the worries may be about it is important that you seek support and help.

Case study 7.1

Jason is a student nurse who due to sickness and a recent family bereavement has fallen behind with his practice hours. Jason is keen to make these hours up as soon as possible on his return to work and arranges to work a couple of shifts in the practice area during each of his allocated theory weeks. Jason becomes tired and feels under pressure. He starts to fall behind with his academic work. In this instance Jason is trying to juggle both the academic demands of his course with the required theory components so as not to fall behind. He becomes stressed and requires further time off sick with exhaustion.

In this situation, Jason should have met with his personal tutor on his initial return from work to develop a plan for making up his clinical hours that ensures he has adequate opportunity for rest. It is important that health and wellbeing conversations are a normal part of student life and you are able to discuss your needs with your personal tutor so that personalised plans can be developed. The university wellbeing team will also be able to signpost you to support and it may be necessary to arrange an appointment with your GP. Ensuring that you have opportunity to stay connected with social support and having opportunity to switch off from the pressures of everyday life is also important. There is evidence to suggest that cognitive behavioural therapy, physical and mental relaxation techniques such as massage and meditation and making organisational changes to increase support and change work schedules can help reduce stress levels (Ruotsalainen et al., 2015).

Other Tools and Strategies to Promote Resilience That You May Have the Opportunity to Engage With

- Many healthcare settings offer structured peer support initiatives such as the allocation of a buddy at the start of shift who can relieve you for breaks and vice versa. Ideally this should be planned by the shift coordinator at the start of the shift.
- Team-building initiatives and events are a good way to meet new colleagues and help build supportive relationships within team and managers. Examples of these include team huddles where the shift team meet to discuss what is happening to improve communication, inclusivity and enable discussions around the challenges faced.
- Many healthcare areas have allocated wellbeing or mental health champions who can be a useful resource for accessing support
- The Advocating for Education and Quality Improvement (A-EQUIP) model and role of the professional Midwifery Advocate (PMA) and Professional Nurse Advocate (PNA) is an employer-led model that facilitates opportunity for clinical supervision and reflection on practice with a view to making improvements (NHS England, 2017, 2021).
- Managing your time and expectations is vital when combining theoretical study with a practical course. This will enable you to maintain a healthy work-life balance while combining academic study with clinical shift work and the pressures this brings. Ensure that you keep a diary and draw up plans to help you manage your deadlines for assessment submission. Remember that while it is important you make the most of opportunities that present themselves, it is also important to say no sometimes to enable you to manage your workload effectively.
- Recognise red flags – when moving from stress to distress. Undertake your emotional health check.
- Developing your resilience toolkit: create a mind-map/build a tool kit

Chapter Summary

In this chapter, we sought to explore the concept of resilience and the factors that inhibit and positively contribute to resilience. We have highlighted some of the situations in healthcare that may test your resilience, and workplace stress is a major factor and stress indicators have been outlined. We have examined the research within the field of resilience and offered resources to help you develop and maintain resilience as a strategy for managing challenges and enhancing emotional wellbeing within the workplace. With the role of caring, having a high emotional toll on individuals together with the stresses of being a student having to meet deadlines both in the theoretical and clinical aspects, building and sustaining your resilience is essential. The strategies and toolkit we have set out are for you to put into action.

8

Building and Maintaining Your Physical Health

Victoria Adebola and
Annette Chowthi-Williams

NMC Standards of Proficiency for Registered Nurses (NMC, 2018)
Professional Standards Social Work England (2019)
Standards of Proficiency (HCPC, 2018)

Nursing & Midwifery Council

This chapter will address the following platforms and proficiencies:

- Being an accountable professional
- Promoting health and preventing ill health
- Improving safety and quality of care

Social Work England

This chapter will address the following standards:

Standard 2: Establish and maintain the trust and confidence of people
Standard 3: Be accountable for the quality of my practice and the decisions I make
Standard 4: Maintain my continuing professional development
Standard 5: Act safely and with professional integrity

Health and Care Professional Council

This chapter will address the following proficiencies:

1 Be able to practise safely and effectively within their scope of practice
3 Be able to maintain fitness to practise
4 Be able to practise as an autonomous professional exercising their own professional judgement
8 Be able to communicate effectively
12 Be able to assure the quality of their practice

Chapter aims

After reading this chapter, you will be able to:

• Understand the impact of physical activities on the body.
• Gain knowledge on the importance of healthy eating and benefits to the body.
• Understand how to develop appropriate supportive social, community and family support.
• Understand the significance of rest, sleep, relaxation, recreation and work-life balance.

Introduction

In this chapter, we want to put the spotlight on your physical health. There is urgency to engage you in caring for yourselves and maintaining your physical health. Your physical health is linked to other aspects of your health and caring for your physical health will have a bearing on your mental, psychological and social health. The chapter will begin with defining health and exploring the potential challenges for health and social care students. We then give you an overview of the impact of physical activity on the anatomy and physiology of the body. Physical health is impacted by a range of sources such as healthy eating, good rest and sleep, a thriving social, community and family support, much relaxation and regular physical activities. We explore how to improve and maintain your physical health. And we guide you through how best to equip yourself with the right resources for continued optimum physical health.

What is Health?

We have discussed in previous chapters that the work of caring takes a high physical toll on the body. You will be engaged in high physical work caring for patients, attending meetings, working with and observing the many professionals in health and social care, whilst working towards your proficiencies in a variety of settings. You will be practising in different environments such as community and primary care which involves covering large geographical areas and GP attached boundaries as we indicated earlier. However, while there is a high physical toll on student's physical health, equally the emotional labour of caring is high and thus maintaining good physical health will contribute to managing the high emotional toll.

Historically, there has been a disconnect around the interplay between physical and mental health which in turns impacts how we manage both. This is because physical and mental health are often viewed as separate entities. However, research indicates that anything that affects the physical body affects mental health. The World Health Organization in 1948 defined health as 'a state of complete physical, mental and social well-being and not merely the absence of disease or infirmity' (WHO, 2021). Although this definition stems from a medicalised model of health, and attempts to view health as holistic encompassing the various components that determines our health and wellbeing, it may be unrealistic and unattainable to always maintain a 'complete state' of health at all times (Huber et al., 2011); conversely, it views health in the physical, mental and social dimensions and acknowledges the relationships between these dimensions and how they are interlinked and important in maintaining your health and wellbeing. It also highlights the socio-economic and environmental factors that determine our health. There is now increasing recognition for everyone particularly healthcare professionals to consider psychological wellbeing when addressing physical health and vice versa (Figure 8.1).

Being a Health and Social Care Student: The Potential Challenges and Solutions

We have highlighted and discussed throughout this book the many potential challenges health and social care students may face. There are growing complexities while undertaking your studies and these might include:

- managing your attendance to lectures, meeting deadlines for assignments and exams
- adjusting emotionally, financially and socially to change

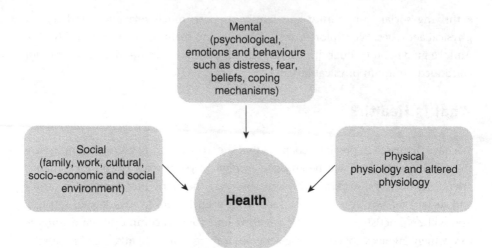

Figure 8.1 The different elements of health

- managing expectations and demands from family members
- managing clinical placement, juggling home life and academic work
- the stress of university life and limited time for other social activities (MacDonald, 2018).

Alongside these issues, student may find they are ill-prepared for the future workforce to deliver high-quality care and manage the pressure of caring for complex and large caseloads linked to increasing patients living with co-morbidities and multi-morbidities. This has led to increase reports of compassion-fatigue, burnout and trauma, high attrition rates and inability to recruit the required numbers of students to grow the workforce (Swift & Twycross, 2020).

A study found that although students were willing to assist during the recent COVID-19 pandemic as a moral duty or to complete their placement in good time, they were unprepared for the impact of separation from family to protect them, challenges with shortage of PPE and inadequate resources, and most significantly the physical and emotional toll on their health and wellbeing (Swift et al., 2020). Students can be adequately prepared for the academic and clinical rigour of the programme through support provided by the academic and clinical teams, develop important skills including planning, time management, organisational skills and realistic expectations about the course and be resilient.

Other protective factors that can encourage continuity and progression on the course include your health and wellbeing, building your resilience and drawing on support from family, friends and peers, practice assessors, supervisors, colleagues in placements, personal tutors and support for the transitioning process (Swift & Twycross, 2020).

You can improve your physical health by maintaining a routine of exercising daily, eating healthy and sleeping well which will in turn impact your mental health positively. You can also improve the social and psychological aspects of work by making small changes that can enable you to build resilience and improve your self-esteem and foster better working relationships with your colleagues at work (Delphis, 2019). We discussed building and maintaining your resilience in Chapter 7.

━━━━━━━━━ ACTIVITY **8.1** ━━━━━━━━━

Reflection

Can you think of a time when you experienced a stressful situation or extreme stress or intense emotion?

Describe this event.

How did this make you feel? What actions did you take to manage the experience and your emotion? Who else was involved?

Was any activity or action particularly helpful? If yes, list them.

Biological Make Up: Physical and Mental Health

Although your genetic makeup or hereditary genetics predisposes you to certain illness, for example mental illness or type 2 diabetes, there is sufficient evidence that some non-biological factors affect the expression of these illnesses. Certain lifestyle factors including limited exercise, excessive alcohol intake, unhealthy eating, sedentary lifestyle, stressful environment and limited social connections can lead to type 2 diabetes, liver diseases, cardiovascular diseases, some cancers and mental illnesses (NHS, 2021).

Individuals who are genetically predisposed to mental illness might become ill when certain psychological factors trigger the genetics. For example, a negative event occurring suddenly or the cumulative effect of negative incidences occurring at different times may impact one's health especially if the negative buffer outweighs the positive one and can result in an acute mental illness. Negative effects could be, for example, experiencing a stressful day at work, a disorganised work environment with no support from the team, working under pressure with limited resources and manpower. The recent COVID-19 pandemic forcing staff to work differently and under stressful conditions may lead to a resentment for the job and the work environment (Delphis, 2019). This may lead reduced sleep, feeling anxious, stress and finally feeling depressed.

Some individuals may start to drink to numb the feeling which may in turn lead to physical illness including liver disease and mental illness such as isolation and depression. A person's mental health can be impacted by a variety of positive or complex and varied negative events. Chronic health conditions such as kidney disease, chronic obstructive pulmonary disease and diabetes increases one's risk of developing mental illness such as depression or anxieties. Similarly, there is a link between depression and coronary heart disease and schizophrenic or being diagnosed with schizophrenia doubles one's risk of death from heart disease and triples the risk of respiratory illness (Mental Health Foundation, 2022). Lifestyle factors are significant influence on physical and mental health. Similarly, someone at risk of type 2 diabetes if eating unhealthily and living a sedentary lifestyle might exacerbate type 2 diabetes early unlike someone who manages their health and exercises and eats well.

SCENARIO 8.1

Lucy is a second-year student nurse. Her current placement is in ICU where she finds 12 and half hour shift very busy and high pace. She finishes work late and is a mother to two young children under 5. When she gets home, she hardly has time to plan and prepare for the next day. So, she eats convenience food and snacks a lot at work.

Lucy notices she is finding it difficult to climb flight of stairs without getting breathless and is struggling with her fitness level and keeping up with her toddler and school age children at home.

ACTIVITY 8.2

Research

What is happening to Lucy?

What actions can Lucy take to improve her physical health?

Is there anyone she can talk to or receive support from?

Make a list of possible people/organisations/?

Benefits of physical activity: exercise

Exercise improves organ function. During exercise, the muscles demand for oxygen increases, similarly, carbon dioxide and metabolic by products such as hydrogen and potassium ions produced by the muscle causes the blood vessels to dilate. This allows more blood to flow in to supply the needed oxygen to the muscles, the heart and lungs and other organs in the body. Taking regular exercise increases blood flow to vital organs and reduces risks of developing high blood pressure, coronary diseases, and some cancers by 25%. Exercise improves the balance of cholesterol by increasing higher levels of HDL cholesterol also known as good cholesterol (BNF, 2022). It is important to eat well and keep hydrated before, during and after exercise.

Regular physical activity also helps in regulating and maintaining the body's optimum weight by helping to balance your intake and output. During exercise, the body uses up energy and excess calories which can help create a healthy energy balance thus preventing obesity and type 2 diabetes, cardiovascular disease and helps keep you fit. Sedentary lifestyle increases the risk of obesity and obesity is a major risk factor for type 2 diabetes. About 3.5 million people in the United Kingdom live with diabetes, with nine in ten of this type 2 diabetes. People living with type 2 diabetes should exercise regularly to help keep their blood glucose levels within the target range, control the body's sensitivity to insulin and lower blood pressure and reduces your chances of developing diabetes-related problems (BNF, 2022).

Improving our physical health activity and physical wellbeing

As already established, sedentary lifestyle increases the dangers of developing physical and mental illnesses. Physical activity contributes to mental wellbeing and thus it is recommended that you:

- Exercising regularly and maintaining your physical activity helps to develop adequate muscles, bones, joints, heart and lung function.
- We start to lose muscle and bones density, but you can help to prevent this by exercising regularly.
- Lifting weights can improve muscles functions and keep bones strong and healthy throughout life to help prevent injury, falls and fractures and osteoporosis.
- Engaging in physical activity can increase bone mineral density and helps to maintain strong bones as we age.
- Moderate aerobic activity, such as walking, swimming and cycling, can help to treat and reduce pain caused by osteoarthritis. It is pertinent to keep the joints moving and perform some strengthening exercises (Puri, 2022).

National Institute of Health. (2021). Physical wellness toolkit. Available at: https://www.nih.gov/health-information/physical-wellness-toolkit#:~:text=6%20strategies%20for%20improving%20your%20physical%20health%201,healthy%20diet.%20...%206%20Build%20healthy%20habits.%20

NHS. (2021). Exercise. Available from: https://www.nhs.uk/live-well/exercise/

Relationship Between Physical Activity and Mental Wellbeing

Physical activity can improve your mental health and wellbeing and regular exercise is good for the mind and the body and can reduce the risk of developing depression and dementia, relieve stress and anxiety, and improve mood. During exercise certain chemicals known as neurotransmitters (dopamine and serotonin) are released in the brain, which are important for one's mood and thinking (BUPA, 2019). Neurotransmitters are substances produced and released by individual nerve cells to communicate with each other by passing across junctions between the cells (synapses), or coordinate communications both within the brain and between the brain and the rest of your body. Adequate neurotransmitters such as serotonin and dopamine are important in maintaining system balance, essential for a healthy brain and optimal brain/mental function, healthy behaviour and decision-making.

Dopamine is mainly responsible for keeping one feeling motivated, deliver a sense of satisfaction when playing sports, learning something new, accomplishing a task or project, or getting a promotion at work. On the other hand, low levels or imbalance of dopamine can result in reduced function of the brain and under activity with symptoms including fatigue, apathy, lack of focus, forgetfulness, mood swings, insomnia, cravings including sugar, reduced motivation and poor motor control (Rowe, 2020).

Serotonin on the other hand is a soothing neurotransmitter produced by the brain, mostly from the amino acid derived from dietary proteins, regulates many transmitter systems and plays a role in the brain and body's ability to communicate, and it is linked with learning and memory. It has been referred to as the 'don't worry, be happy' neurotransmitter. Serotonin helps maintain a balanced mood, boosts self-confidence, supports a healthy appetite, decreasing worries and concerns, facilitates deep sleep and enables survival functions like temperature regulation and breathing. Signs of serotonin deficiency include fluctuation between low mood and overexcited mood, changes in gut health and appetite. Low serotonin activity can result in reduced mental alertness, carbohydrate cravings and binge eating, digestive and other intestinal problems, sleep issues, feeling overwhelmed and unhappy, headaches, anger and irritability. Serotonin can be maintained by eating the healthy balanced meals that facilitate serotonin production (Rowe, 2020).

Depending on your clinical placement and how busy it is, it is important to:

- reduce time spent sitting down.
- break up long periods of not moving with some activity to reduce your risk of developing cardiovascular disease.
- keep the physical activity going during your days off, it is advisable to walk when you can and avoid driving short distances.
- find ways to incorporate activities within your daily schedule. The guideline is for adult to engage in at least 150 minutes of moderate intensity activity weekly and or 75 minutes vigorous intensity exercise weekly and to engage in strengthening exercise to work the essential muscles such as gardening and weights at least twice weekly.

Eating for Good Physical Health

Good nutrition or balanced meals influence the way we feel, our body's development, management and prevention of numerous physical and mental health illnesses including depression and Alzheimer's. A healthy balanced diet should include the right proportion of macronutrients such as proteins (important for the normal growth and maintenance of the body), essential fats (the body with energy and essential fatty acids), complex carbohydrates (provides energy for the body), and micronutrients including vitamins, minerals and water which are essential for the body to function adequately, however required in smaller amounts. Macronutrients are divided into the fat-soluble vitamins such as vitamins A, D, E and K and water-soluble vitamins which are vitamin B's, folate and vitamin C. Most of these vitamins can be obtained from food except vitamin D due to reduced sunlight in the United Kingdom (BNF, 2022).

Approximately 1 in 5 people have low vitamin D levels (serum levels < 25 nmol/l). Inadequate vitamin D levels may be associated with a higher risk of poor bone and muscle health, increased risk of conditions such as rickets in children and osteomalacia in adults falls poor muscle strength. The Scientific Advisory Committee on Nutrition (SACN) recommends everyone aged 4 and above to take a supplement of 10 µg (micrograms)/day; 8.5–10 µg/day for infants and younger children. This is particularly important for dark-skinned people where the melanin in the skin can affect the absorption of vitamin D (BNF, 2022).

Eating well adds years to your life, improve your skin, energy levels, moods and prevent diseases. The Long-Term Plan (2019) for the nation's health sets out strategies for tacking many of the diseases that are currently impacting our health.

Lucy enjoys her comfort food, pastries cakes and take away during placement. She is noticing her uniform is tighter, and struggles to perform certain task without being breathless and feels lethargic.

- Describe what is happening to Lucy?
- Describe why this is happening?
- What happens to the body when you consume high sugary meals or drinks?
- What portion of macronutrients should she consume daily?
- What can Lucy do and who can she talk to?

As students you could eat healthily and maintain good eating habits by:

- preparing and planning your meals and incorporating healthy meal options.
- avoiding simple sugars found in pastries, cakes and some carbohydrates that may lead to spikes in your insulin level.

- avoiding high fatty foods that may lead to high cholesterol.
- consider opting for brown bread and pastas and dietary (non-digestible carbohydrates) in your diet as their benefit include reducing the risk of some diseases including heart disease, type 2 diabetes and colon cancer and it is beneficial for your digestive health and reduces the risk of constipation (BNF, 2022; NHS, 2019).
- eat more plant base food, chickpeas, lentils, kidney beans, nuts, vegetable, fruits and fish.
- cut down on red meat and processed meats and foods.

Eat more of these foods

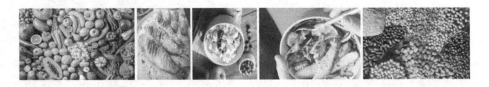

Figure 8.2　Foods that are beneficial for health

Eat less of these foods

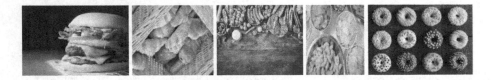

Figure 8.3　Foods that impact your health negatively

Hydration for Good Physical Health

Water makes up 60% of body weight in men and 50–55% in women and it is important in regulating temperature, transporting nutrients and compounds in blood, removing waste products that are passed in the urine and acting as a lubricant and shock absorber in joints. Dehydration can affect one's mental and physical health. Symptoms of mild dehydration include a dry mouth, headaches and poor concentration. The amount of fluid required may vary based on the weather, the amount of one's physical activity and your age. The average recommendation is 6–8 glasses of fluid daily. To prevent being dehydrated especially during the warmer months, it is important to drink fluid regularly particularly during busy shifts in placement. You can have teas and coffees but limit the coffees because of the effect of caffeine which is a stimulant (BNF, 2022).

━━━━━━━━ **ACTIVITY 8.3** ━━━━━━━━

Research and Reflection

Lucy does not enjoy drinking water. She prefers fizzy drinks and drinks a bottle of coke during a 11.5-hour shift. By the end of the shift, she experiences this: her lips are dry, and her skin is starting to show signs of being dry, she is feeling lethargic and sometimes feels lightheaded. She is also drinking over 5 units of alcohol after every shift.

Describe what is happening to Lucy?

Describe why this is happening?

What happens when you consume too little fluids?

What type of drinks will you advice?

What can Lucy do and who can she talk to?

Sleep and Rest for Good Physical Health

It is important to rest well and have a sleep routine. Plan and organise your day and activities so it does not interfere with your sleep and rest. During your off days, take time to rest and recuperate from the long shift patter and nights.

Benefits of sleep and rest include:

- immune system boost
- improves memory
- concentration and productivity
- your health restores and good sleep stimulates creativity
- helps with weight management as you do not binge eat and consume less calories
- keeps you mentally and emotionally fit
- it slows down the aging process and makes you happier
- healthy and glowing skin

10 rules to get your body ready for good sleep

- Set a wake-up time
- Exercise
- Get outdoors
- Eat less before bed
- Have caffeine in the mornings only

- Meditate
- Avoid regular alcohol in the evenings
- Quit smoking and if challenging cut out smoking in the evening
- Read a book, listen to music and avoid screen activity
- Get into the habit of seeing bed as a place to sleep, i.e. avoid spending time in the bedroom during the day

(Read more and the research – *Daily Mail*, Monday, 17 January 2022)

━━━━━ ACTIVITY 8.4 ━━━━━

Research and Reflection

Can you think of times when you could not sleep well?

Make a list of the impact on your physical and mental health

Now compare your findings with those in the link belowhttps://www.sleepfoundation.org/sleep-deprivation

Family, Social Support and Work-Life Balance for Good Physical Health

According to Maslow's hierarchy of needs, after your basic needs (nutrition, hydration and shelter) are met the next most important needs are social needs and indicators of social determinant of health that influences health outcomes. Everyone yearns to belong somewhere or to be connected to people (Thomas, Liu, & Umberson, 2017). Family and friends are a strong support network. It is important to stay connected and find time to spend with one's support network. This means you will be able to be supported through the academic stresses and any challenging times ahead.

━━━━━ ACTIVITY 8.5 ━━━━━

Reflection

Can you identify your sources of social and family support?

Do you feel and think you have sufficient support from these sources?

Where else could you get social support?

Strong relationship and connections increase one's quality of life. Good support system can help you make better decisions around healthy living. Family relationships and support has a bearing on the health and wellbeing of individuals, including emotional health and equipping us with the resources to deal with the range of challenges expected. The lack of family support has psychological impacts and may contribute to individuals becoming more vulnerable to stresses (Parra et al., 2018; Rodriguez, 2018). A Harvard study which started in 1938 and thought to be one of the world's longest studies of adult life to determine childhood experiences on midlife health and wellbeing showed that participants who enjoyed better health and lived longer were the those who leaned into relationships, with family, with friends, with community (Harvard Second Generation Study) https://www.a-dultdevelopmentstudy.org/2nd-generation-study.

Excessive and sustained stress can lead to prolonged levels of cortisol in the bloodstream and have negative effects including impacting blood sugar balances such as hyperglycaemia, high blood pressure, impaired cognitive performance, increased abdominal fat, lowered immunity and inflammatory responses in the body and other health consequences (Thau, Gandhi, & Sharma, 2022). Cortisol, also known as the 'stress hormone', is produced by the adrenal glands and it is important in the way the body responds to or manages stressful situations. It is therefore important that when you are feeling stressed to speak to your practice assessors or supervisors in placements. Your personal tutor is also a source of support. Your university will have wellbeing or student support team to help manage these stressful conditions. It is important to also recognise these triggers. Practicing mindfulness can be helpful and other therapies offered by professionals.

In placement, for example, you may experience challenging events with colleagues, the team or with patients, service users or clients. In this kind of situation, your practice assessor should be able to support you or conduct a debriefing with you. There is also support available through the healthcare trust and your universities.

Chapter Summary

We focused a number of chapters on your holistic health and wellbeing. In this chapter we delved in a little detail on your physical health. You will have understood having read and undertaken the activities in the chapter that physical health and mental are interlinked. The role of a health and social care student is a demanding one as we have consistently discussed through this book. It can be physically exhausting, and thus taking care of your physical health is essential. Thus, healthy eating, keeping yourself hydrated, having plenty of rest and sleep and taking care of your mental health is a must. Regular exercise, meditation, mindfulness and eating well, social support and balancing family and work, should enable you to manage both aspects of your study, the theoretical and practice elements. It is essential that you make every effort to adopt the advice and support made available in this chapter to improve and maintain your physical health.

9

Strategies and Tools for Enhancing Your Wellbeing

Janet Goddard and
Annette Chowthi-Williams

NMC Standards of Proficiency for Registered Nurses (NMC, 2018)
Professional Standards Social Work England (2019)
Standards of Proficiency (HCPC, 2018)

Nursing & Midwifery Council

This chapter will address the following platforms and proficiencies:

1 Being an accountable professional
2 Promoting health and preventing ill health

Social Work England

This chapter will address the following standards:

Standard 3: Be accountable for the quality of my practice and the decisions I make
Standard 4: Maintain my continuing professional development
Standard 5: Act safely and with professional integrity

Health and Care Professional Council

This chapter will address the following proficiencies:

1 Be able to practise safely and effectively within their scope of practice
3 Be able to maintain fitness to practise
4 Be able to practise as an autonomous professional, exercising their own professional judgement
11 Be able to reflect on and review practice
12 Be able to assure the quality of their practice

Chapter aims

After reading this chapter, you will be able to:

- Describe the relationship between mental and physical health.
- Identify strategies for self-care and support.
- Understand what is needed to maintain physical and mental health.
- Demonstrate an awareness of the issues relating to mental and physical health.

Introduction

In this chapter, we are creating some additional resources to enhance and maintain your wellbeing. We begin by reminding you that health needs to be viewed holistically and not to be separated into different components. We then continue the chapter with physical, mental, psychological and emotional health and the additional strategies and tools that you can access. There are three areas of health concern that we need to pay attention to in this chapter mainly because these are habits that can be challenging to manage and needs to be managed because of the impacts on our health and wellbeing. These are alcohol, smoking and obesity. We provide you with tools, resources and activities that you can access. Throughout this chapter, we refer to other chapters in this book where you can also find available resources so that you feel equipped to engage with your personal and professional growth and development.

Our Holistic Health and Wellbeing

In many of the chapters in this book, we have indicated the importance of your mental, emotional, psychological, physical and social health and wellbeing. These different aspects of the individual are all interconnected and thus improving one aspect of health will help improve the other. For example, improving our physical health will improve our mental, emotional and psychological health. We explored the mind, consciousness and emotions and their links in Chapter 4 where we stressed the importance of understanding these connections. There are many factors that can have an impact on our mind and behaviour and thus impact how we think, act and feel.

Physical health

We know that physical activity is an important element of achieving a sense of wellbeing, and organisations such as MIND promote it to improve your mental health. When we think of physical health, we sometimes think it means strenuous exercise, such as running, but it is better to consider it as engaging with moving ourselves physically rather than sitting around engaging in non-physical or sedentary activities, such as watching television or using technology in some form. Weiler et al. (2013) recognise that physical activity correlates positively with health, and affective, social and cognitive function, so it is understandable that if physical inactivity has been the experience in childhood, it may also still be the experience in adulthood. The effects, however, might be more noticeable, such as sleep problems or depressive symptoms (Stea, Solaas, & Kleppang, 2022). It is possible to understand why we need to address any inactivity as the effects can be significant.

Try to do the activity below but recognise that if you have not been exercising for a longer period of time, it might take a while to build up your fitness to a level where you can engage for longer. You should be able to see a change in yourself over a period of time, such as better sleep, or better engagement with your studies, but you might also find that you start to build friendships with like-minded individuals, and you can then encourage each other to continue and become fitter together.

━━━━━━━━ **ACTIVITY 9.1** ━━━━━━━━

Choose one activity from the list below and do it for 1 week. Slowly add in another activity or do the one you originally chose for longer.

- Brisk walking
- Water aerobics
- Riding a bike
- Dancing
- Tennis
- Take the stairs
- Running
- Swimming
- Skipping
- Play football, rugby, netball

https://www.nhs.uk/live-well/exercise/exercise-guidelines/physical-activity-guidelines-for-adults-aged-19-to-64/

Image: https://openclipart.org/detail/222008/woman-exercising-silhouette

---

If you have a disability, that does not prevent you from exercising, but it can have other challenges able-bodied individuals might not experience, such as poorly equipped gyms or buildings that are not easily accessible. Nonetheless, we need to think more positively about what you can do as there are a significant number of exercises available to you.

ACTIVITY 9.2

Think about what you can do from the list below, and again, build up slowly and do not push yourself beyond what is comfortable. You might also wish to speak with your GP first.

- Wheelchair basketball
- Seated knee-raise
- Swimming
- Sit to stand
- Seated triceps dips
- Seated shoulder press
- Reverse crunches
- Resistance band exercises

If you are a little concerned, watch the videos below to help guide you, you can also form a group or do you have another person you like to exercise with?
https://www.disabledliving.co.uk/blog/sports-activities-for-people-with-disabilities/
https://disabilityhorizons.com/2016/10/top-10-exercises-disabled-people/https://www.activenorfolk.org/public/get-active/active-at-home/disability-exercises/

Image: http://www.freepngclipart.com/free-png/70837-summer-basketball-cycling-esportes-paralympic-sports-games

Mental and psychological health

Many of us recognise that there are times when, although we are generally well mentally, we have periods of time when we feel more fragile. It might be external pressure, such as the pressure of study, assessments, or work, or it might be internal pressures, such as stress, fear or mental fatigue. Where we are in our mental state often is evidenced in how we respond to the world around us. There are natural highs and lows in life and, as a rule, we are able to respond accordingly, but on occasion, we are not able to do it, and we become overwhelmed, tearful or withdraw from those around us. The feeling may pass without too much effort from us but, sometimes, we need to be more proactive in resolving the issues we are dealing with (Hallam et al., 2018). If we just leave it, we risk it developing into a more serious problem, one that is far harder to resolve, so the sooner we address it, the better it is for us, even if it is painful to begin with.

We are not always willing to speak about our mental health as we recognise that there is sometimes a stigma that attaches to it, and so we remain silently spiralling downwards. The World Health Organization launched a Special Initiative for Mental Health in 2019, in which it recognises depression as one of the leading causes of disability and yet, although treatment for it is low cost, we do not seek access to it. Often, we prefer not to speak about how we are feeling and feel that it is a sign of weakness to reveal this side of ourselves, but that prevents us engaging fully with the support that is around us and creating change for ourselves. The Mental Health Foundation have a free download (How to ... mental health.pdf) which is useful to begin the process of understanding your mental health and recognising its impact on your overall wellbeing and alongside offering tips and guidance, it aims to make us invest in ourselves, which we do not often do, so why not download it and start the journey back to good mental health.

━━━━━━━━━━ **ACTIVITY 9.3** ━━━━━━━━━━

Reflection

Look at the Worry Tree and try to think of something you are worried about. Follow the guidance in the diagram to see whether this is a strategy you can use to deal with future concerns.

Butler and Hope (1995) The Worry Tree. Accessed via https://positivepsychology. com/mental-health-exercises-interventions/

Critical Thinking

- Did you apply your problem properly?
- Did you really consider whether you could resolve it by following the instructions above?
- What could you have done differently?
- Will you use it again in future, or have you found another way in this book that was more useful?

Signposting

Student Hub

Check whether your university has either a Student Hub, or a similar team as it is where you can access a range of different support services, including support for a range of disability and mental health conditions. Some also have links to allow you to access support for Disabled Students Allowance (DSA) and Individual Support Plans (ISP), which your Course Leader will be sent so they understand what support you might need on your course, and they can speak with other lecturers teaching you to ensure they understand your specific requirements. You might also find the Government link helpful, as it will allow you to see what support is available to you as a disabled student.

Further information regarding DSA from https://www.gov.uk/disabled-students-allowance-dsa

Wellbeing

The Wellbeing Team at your university are a team dedicated to ensuring that you have equal access to your course and to the other facilities available to you at your university. They can support you with any physical, mental or communication barriers you may have in accessing your course. Universities are committed to ensuring you have access to the facilities and the campuses so that your engagement and learning are not negatively impacted.

Welfare

The Welfare Team are available to offer you support with any personal or emotional problems, so that you do not have to address things alone or without support. You might find you can access them as part of the Wellbeing Team, but they might be a separate body too. Do check, as they offer another layer of support to you.

We recognise that there are times you might need more urgent or immediate support, so please find additional numbers here for you to contact.

> **The Samaritans** – 116 123 (24 hours)
> **NHS Direct** – 111 (the NHS non-emergency number)
> **Non-Emergency Police** – 101
> **Emergency Services** – **999** (Fire, Police or Ambulance)
> **Frank** – (advice and support if you are worried about drug misuse) 0300 123 6600/Text: 82111, or, talk to Frank via talktofrank.com
> **Nightline** – (a confidential and anonymous listening service run by students for students). Contact them on 020 7631 0101 (6 pm to 8 am – every night of term), or via nightline.org.uk

Debt Advice – (a confidential advice service if you are worried about loans, credit and debt) 0800 043 40 50 Freephone (Monday to Friday 8 am to 8 pm, Saturday 9 am to 3 pm), or via debtadvicefoundation.org

Refuge – (Support for people fleeing violence and abuse) – 0808 2000 247 (24 hours) or refuge.org.uk

Money advice

You can get help and support with your money as we recognise this can be a source of worry and stress to you. If you need support, please contact the Student Advice at your university, as they will be able to guide you in who to contact.

Study support

We recognise that some students are concerned that they will not be able to engage properly with academic study and academic writing, so universities have addressed this by having a team dedicated to Study Support. They are there to help you with all aspects of how you write and engage with your academic learning, so please speak with your student services who will guide you appropriately.

Care leaver support

You can access support from application to graduation, to support you through your life at university. UCAS recognise the help you might require, so please engage with them via this link to see what is available to you https://www.ucas.com/undergraduate/applying-university/individual-needs/ucas-undergraduate-care-experienced-students

Careers advice

Universities have a Careers' Advice Team to support you into work after graduating. They can help you with creating your CV, job applications, interview preparation, part-time work during your studies, and volunteer positions, right up to preparing for your graduate career, so do please contact them if this would be helpful to you.

There is further support for our international students, so contact your student services to seek guidance and support around issues such as accommodation, finance, Visas, but also, information around studying with your chosen university.

Student advice

If you are experiencing financial difficulties or funding problems, or you have any questions about money, please contact your Student Advice service, as they can help to consider and resolve your financial difficulties.

Student Union

Your Student Union is there to support you, and you can access them directly. The range of services they offer is significant, so do make contact with the Student Union active at your chosen university. You might also wish to join them, which means you can become proactive in helping other students too.

Emotional Health

We explored emotions in some depth in Chapters 4, 5 and 6 and we learnt that our two minds emotional and cognitive are interlinked and work in harmony with each other. We provided you with activities and resources to manage your emotions. You may have experienced the power of emotions and at times struggled with managing your emotions. You may find yourself experiencing a range of emotions whilst undertaking your professional health and social care course.

In university, you may feel anxiety at the share volume of work, having to grapple with new ideas or before an exam. Fear, apprehension and panic may be experienced as you approach going into the clinical setting. When you begin to care for patients, service users and clients who are ill, recovering from surgery or receiving treatment for cancer, you may experience a raft of emotions from anticipation to admiration of your patients and how they are coping. As you adjust to change, you may experience a mixture of emotions fear, anxiety, apprehension, joy and feel optimist about your future caring for people. There may be other emotions coming to the surface as you face new challenges.

When faced with these challenges, individuals may feel overwhelmed and tempted to resort to activities that they feel might give them comfort. You may well know of individuals who have turned to alcohol, overeating, smoking or taking drugs. But these strategies may seem beneficial at the time but on a regular basis they have serious impacts on our holistic health. Research has suggested that a little red wine may be good for the heart as is dark chocolate and coffee. But these foods need to be taken in moderation alongside the many activities we have set out in this book.

Alcohol

Some studies have reported benefits of alcohol, particularly red wine, in reducing one's risk of developing heart disease and ischemic stroke, diabetes; it plays a protective role against oxidative stress, reduces cardiovascular risk factors in AHC, and enhances its antioxidant effects with parallel increase of vitamin E, but they have also argued that this should be taken in moderation (Apostolidou et al., 2015; Mayo Clinic, 2021). The NHS guideline for women and men is 14 units a week. Drinking over the recommended guideline can lead to both short-term and long-term risks to the body. Short-term risks of alcohol binging include predisposition to reckless behaviour, crime and being a victim of abuse when inhibitions are down, accidents and injuries violent behaviour, engaging in unprotected sex and as a consequence developing STIs, alcohol poisoning. Long-term consequences of persistent alcohol abuse include depression and anxiety, addiction, liver disease including hepatitis and cirrhosis, cardiovascular disease, stroke and cancers (NHS, 2018; NHS, 2021).

━━━━━━━━ **ACTIVITY 9.4** ━━━━━━━━

Research and Critical Thinking

Sylvia is experiencing stress at work and finding it difficult to cope with the increasing workload and pressures at work. She is also worried about her career progression. Previously, she drank once a week but she is now drinking every evening and more after every shift.

Describe what is happening to Sylvia.

Describe why this is happening and how she is feeling.

What happens to the body when you consume excessive alcohol?

What is the daily recommended consumption?

What test can Sylvia take to determine whether she is drinking over the limit?

What can Sylvia do and who can she talk to?

Support available that can be sought

GP/OH at work
   Your family, friends, peers on your course
   Counselling and talking therapies
   Drink line – 0300 123 1110
   Alcoholics Anonymous (AA) helpline – 0800 9177 650
   Al-Anon Family Groups helpline – 0800 0086 811
   We Are With You for over 50s' – 0808 8010 750
   Adfam – a national charity working with families affected by drugs and alcohol
   The National Association for Children of Alcoholics (Nacoa) – 0800 358 3456
   SMART Recovery groups
   Alcohol Change UK

Resources

NHS Alcohol units – https://www.nhs.uk/live-well/alcohol-advice/calculating-alcohol-units/

Alcohol use disorders identification test (AUDIT) – https://assets.publishing.service.gov.uk/government/uploads/system/uploads/attachment_data/file/684823/Alcohol_use_disorders_identification_test__AUDIT_.pdf

Alcohol use disorders identification test – consumption (AUDIT C) – https://assets.publishing.service.gov.uk/government/uploads/system/uploads/attachment_data/file/684826/Alcohol_use_disorders_identification_test_for_consumption__AUDIT_C_.pdf

NHS Alcohol Support – https://www.nhs.uk/live-well/alcohol-advice/alcohol-support/

NHS Local Support – https://www.nhs.uk/nhs-services/find-alcohol-addiction-support-services/

Talking therapies and counselling – https://www.nhs.uk/mental-health/talking-therapies-medicine-treatments/talking-therapies-and-counselling/benefits-of-talking-therapies/

Obesity

A recent report research report published on 16 March 2022, outlined the data on obesity. According to the report, 28% of adults in England are obese and a further 36% are overweight. In the age group 45–74, the figure was three quarters of people in England. You may not be in any of these categories, but we know that being overweight puts individuals at risk of many diseases and impact their life in many other ways. These diseases include heart diseases and cancers. It is essential to eat the right foods; and in Chapter 8, we gave ideas of foods that you should eat more of and foods to eat less.

Read more on this health challenge in the report below

https://commonslibrary.parliament.uk/research-briefings/sn03336/

What losing half a stone (7 pounds) does for your health (*The Times*, 2022)

- You will sleep better
- It will protect your joints
- Your lung function will be better
- Your sex life will improve
- Back pain will be relieved
- You will find running faster easier
- You will stabilise your body's blood sugar levels
- Your risk of heart disease will be reduced
- Your blood pressure will be lowered
- You will lower the risk of certain types of cancer

7 ways to drops and keep them off

- Create an eating window. As well as cutting calories, eating a late breakfast contributes to the body fasting longer. Eat earlier in the evening. Late eating after 10 pm before going to bed, raises blood sugar levels

- Eat dark berries every day – these boost health and help to shed weight by blasting fat in thighs
- Eat a dollop or two of plain yogurt every day, it wards off hunger and makes it harder for the body to absorb fat from foods
- Eat more fermented foods as its good for gut health and the microbiome regulates metabolism
- If you need to snack, have nuts
- Get one extra hour's sleep at night
- Lift weight or use exercise bands three times a week

(Read the research and full article – *The Times Saturday*, 30 April 2022)

Further support

Slim world – https://www.slimmingworld.co.uk/
    Weight Watchers – https://www.weightwatchers.com/uk/
    Weight loss support groups – https://www.nhs.uk/service-search/other-services/Weight%20loss%20support%20groups/LocationSearch/1429

Smoking

Smoking has been shown to impact both mental and physical health. Studies suggest that people suffering from depression and schizophrenia are twice or thrice as likely to smoke as other people. Although people with mental illness believe that smoking relieves their symptoms, but these effects are only short-term (NHS, 2021). Dopamine, the chemical neurotransmitter made in the brain that supports neurological and physiological functioning, motor function, mood, and even our decision-making, also influences positive feelings and is strongly associated with pleasure and reward. It is often released when the brain is expecting a reward, for example when the brain associates certain activity (food, sex, shopping) with pleasure, this may raise dopamine levels. However, it has been found to be deficient in people with depression (Rowe, 2020). Nicotine contained in cigarettes interferes with dopamine produced in the brain. Although, Nicotine temporarily increases the levels of dopamine in the brain, however, it switches off the brain's natural mechanism to produce dopamine, and over a period of time, this can lead to a feeling or craving for more nicotine to achieve this positive sensation (NHS Inform, 2022).

Smoking is a leading cause of COPD. In the United Kingdom, around 3 million people have COPD, with 2 million undiagnosed (NICE, 2011). The tar from cigarettes irritates and inflames the bronchial tubes, leading to unusual mucus production within the lining of the airway to trap the irritant. This results in a thickened and narrowed airway, clogged and consequently, reducing the air flow through the airways. COPD affects breathing and affects physical and mental health. Quitting smoking improves breathing, energy, improved sex life and fertility, smell and taste, makes you feel less stressed and live longer and protects your family and friends (NICE, 2011). Additional support for quitting smoking can be found on NHS Quit Smoking: https://www.nhs.uk/live-well/quit-smoking/

━━━━━━━━ **ACTIVITY 9.5** ━━━━━━━━

Research and Critical Thinking

Ahmed is now smoking 30–40 cigarettes daily. He has noticed he is coughing more and is worse at night. He is experiencing breathlessness and stops to rest after every 50 yards.

Describe what is happening to Ahmed.

Describe why this is happening and how he is feeling.

What happens to the body when you smoke?

What are the consequences of smoking?

What can Ahmed do and who can he talk to?

Support

GP/OH at work/Her family
  Counselling and talking therapies
  NHS Smokefree helpline – 0300 123 1044.

Resources

NHS Health Risk of smoking – https://www.nhs.uk/common-health-questions/lifestyle/what-are-the-health-risks-of-smoking/
  NICE (2021) Chronic obstructive pulmonary disease in adults https://www.nice.org.uk/guidance/qs10/chapter/introduction
  NHS Quit Support – https://www.nhs.uk/better-health/quit-smoking/

There is support available for all of students throughout their time at university, so please do consider what support you need and access it directly. Remember, your university will work with you throughout your course and support you in becoming an independent and autonomous student. It would be useful to you to identify what support you need from your university so that they can work in partnership with you in developing yourself professionally and personally. Think also about engaging with your physical, mental, emotional and psychological health and become proactive in improving how you are feeling. In partnership with those around you, you can work towards developing yourself personally, so that you become more effective professionally.

Chapter Summary

We wanted to create some additional resources for you to enhance and maintain your wellbeing. In this chapter we reminded you that health needs to be viewed holistically and not to be put into different boxes. We explored the additional strategies and tools that you can access for your physical, mental, psychological and emotional health. We wanted to address three areas of health concern that need attention. These were alcohol, smoking and obesity. These health problems can be challenging to manage and we are keen that you managed these if they are impacting your health and wellbeing. We provided you with tools, resources and activities that you can access and referred you to other chapters where you can also find available resources. With the range of resources at your disposal, you can engage with your personal wellbeing, growth and development.

10

Your Personal Wellbeing Journal

Annette Chowthi-Williams and Team

NMC Standards of Proficiency for Registered Nurses (NMC, 2018)
Professional Standards Social Work England (2019)
Standards of Proficiency (HCPC, 2018)

Nursing & Midwifery Council

This chapter will address the following platforms and proficiencies:

1 Being an accountable professional
2 Promoting health and preventing ill health
5 Leading and managing nursing care and working in teams
6 Improving safety and quality of care
7 Coordinating care

Social Work England

This chapter will address the following standards:

Standard 1: Promote the rights, strengths and wellbeing of people, families and communities

Standard 3: Be accountable for the quality of my practice and the decisions I make

Standard 4: Maintain my continuing professional development

Standard 5: Act safely and with professional integrity

Health and Care Professional Council

This chapter will address the following proficiencies:

1   Be able to practise safely and effectively within their scope of practice
3   Be able to maintain fitness to practise
5   Be aware of the impact of culture, equality and diversity on practice
8   Be able to communicate effectively
9   Be able to work appropriately with others
11   Be able to reflect on and review practice
12   Be able to assure the quality of their practice
13   Understand the key concepts of the knowledge base relevant to their profession
14   Be able to draw on appropriate knowledge and skills to inform practice

---

Chapter aims

After reading this chapter, you will be able to:

- Understand the importance of having a personal wellbeing plan.
- Acquire knowledge of how to assess your health and wellbeing.
- Gain understanding of how to achieve your goals.
- Understand and know how to create and maintain your personal wellbeing plan.

Introduction

In this final chapter, we are keen to show you how to set out, implement and monitor your own personal wellbeing through creating your own journal. The 'one size' fits all approach does not work for everyone. The first step in your personal wellbeing plan is to assess your current state of personal wellbeing and we have provided you with an assessment tool to do so. Once you have completed this, you will gain a picture of the level of your own personal wellbeing. Using this evidence of your present wellbeing, you can then take the next step of setting an action plan to improve your personal wellbeing. We have created an example to illustrate how you can go about setting your goals and steps to achieve your goals. Whilst implementing your action plan, you could regularly monitor and review your progress and if need be, re-set new goals. We will set out resources for you to access which will help to improve and maintain your wellbeing whilst on your studies and beyond.

Making Personal Change

How to manage personal change for the workforce has not been researched greatly in healthcare, though there is information on particular interventions for patients.

> https://www.cochranelibrary.com/about/about-cochrane-reviews
> https://www.nice.org.uk/

It is not easy to bring about change whether it's personal or professional. Many people find themselves starting off making a change but then it becomes a real challenge continuing that change. There are no easy answers about how to go about making a personal change but there are many tools that can help you get started and continue on the path of sustaining your change. We have set out many strategies, tools and resources throughout this book to help you but here are a few more tips:

- Think about what would motivate you to change, e.g. health at risk, your family, inner aspiration, work, wanting to feel and look healthy, saving money, a big social event or supporting a charity. These are only a few ideas but there are many more.
- Try to make small changes first and then step by step. A big change can seem overwhelming.
- When you begin your personal change programme, have in place a support network that can keep you motivated, e.g. friends, family or an activity group.
- Let people around you know that you are embarking on personal change, so that they can support you.
- Chose a role model to help motivate you.
- Give yourself positive feedback regularly.
- Set yourself weekly targets and your overall target.
- As with any change, you will face setbacks, be prepared for these and have a plan in place to get back on track.
- Think about your emotions. What impact do they have on your efforts to make personal change?
- What impact does your thoughts have on your plan for personal change?
- Think about how you might get yourself ready for personal change.

Assessing Your Personal Wellbeing

In order for you to set out a plan to improve and maintain your wellbeing, you have to first assess the current state of your personal wellbeing. This involves undertaking an assessment of:

- your physical health
- your psychological health
- your social health
- your financial health

This is a very straightforward activity. You will see below a guide to assessing and interpreting the results of your holistic health and wellbeing. Please answer these to the best of your ability. You can answer in words, pictures/images or just put a tick.

Rating your wellbeing: Traffic Light and Star rating explained

These are ways of rating your present wellbeing. You can do so through a Star Rating or Colour Code using the Traffic Light System.

Star rating

**** Good
*** Satisfactory
** Poor

Traffic light system

Green: Good
Amber: Satisfactory
Red: Poor

Interpreting star rating or traffic light system

Good/Green means continuing with current plans for your personal wellbeing and review as and when necessary.

Satisfactory/Amber means that you will need to take action on your personal wellbeing. You will need to adjust or create a new plan for improvement of your personal wellbeing and implement the new plan.

Poor/Red means that you will need to take action urgently on your wellbeing. You will need to devise a new plan for improvement of your wellbeing and implement the new plan, including contacting your GP if necessary (Figures 10.1 and 10.2).

Star rating or Traffic light system	Exercise	Rest & relaxation	Eating	Hydration	Sleep	Alcohol intake daily	My BMI & Blood Pressure
Green or ***	I am exercising daily	I have plenty of rest daily & I meditate/ undertake mindfulness/ yoga/ relaxation daily/weekly	I eat on time and I eat plenty of oily fish, vegetables & fruits	I carry a water bottle & refill it regularly. I have tea but limit my coffee intake	I get 7–8 hours sleep every night	I have 2–3 small glasses of wine or 2 pints of larger a week	My BP is 120/80 My BMI is 22
Amber or **	I exercise 2–3 times a week	I do get some rest each week, but I don't meditate/ undertake any relaxation	I eat on time generally and I do have some healthy foods but mostly I have meats fried foods, & sweet foods	I drink when I remember to do so. I do prefer coffee/tea mostly	I get good sleep some nights but I toss and turn a lot. Generally, I get about 5–6 hours sleep each night	I have 2 large glasses of wine or 2 pints of larger daily	My BP is 130/90 My BMI 25
Red or *	I do little or no exercise	I am too busy to rest and relax	I grab food when I can. I prefer pre-prepared meals and plenty of sweet foods to keep my energy levels up	I grab a coffee/ tea/hot cocoa every now and then	I toss & turn every night. Eventually, I get about 4–5 hours sleep. I am usually very tired most days	I have 2–3 large glasses of wine or larger every day. More at the weekends more	My BP is 145/90 My BMI is 30

Figure 10.1 Assessing My Physical Health: Abesola

How am I feeling at home/work today and what am I thinking	Write down your thoughts and feeling when at home/work or and Attach emoji of your thoughts and feelings Draw your own picture of your feelings and thoughts
How am I feeling at university today and what am I thinking	Write down your thoughts and feeling when attending university to undertake your modules or and Attach emoji of your thoughts and feelings Draw your own picture of your feelings and thoughts
How am I feeling in clinical practice and what am I thinking	Write down your thoughts and feeling when you are practice or and Attach emoji of your thoughts and feelings Draw your own picture of your feelings and thoughts

Figure 10.2 Assessing My Psychological Health: Abesola

How am I feeling as I am writing up my assignment and what am I thinking?	Write down your thoughts and feeling when you have to work on assignments and prepare for exams or and Attach emoji of your thoughts and feelings Draw your own picture of your feelings and thoughts
How am I feeling with assignment /exam deadline pending and what am I thinking?	Write down your thoughts and feeling when you have assignment/exam deadlines to meet or and Attach emoji of your thoughts and feelings Draw your own picture of your feelings and thoughts
How am I feeling with the support am getting and what am I thinking?	Write down your thoughts and feeling when you have assignment/exam deadlines to meet or and Attach emoji of your thoughts and feelings Draw your own picture of your feelings and thoughts

Figure 10.2 Assessing My Psychological Health: Abesola (*Continued*)

Table 10.1 Interpreting my psychological health

GREEN ***	Feeling happy and satisfied with life Looking forward and enjoying the course/lectures/activities Looking forward to going into practice and working with my colleagues Keen to be with my group I enjoy researching and writing up my assignment I am ahead with my assignment work and on target to meet the deadlines Feeling great with the support I am getting
AMBER **	Feeling life is tough and I am not satisfied with the direction of my life I anxious/unhappy about attending lectures I am not looking forward to going into practice I am experiencing low moods during lectures and on placement, even at home I am finding it a challenge to focus on most things I am constantly thinking about assignment deadlines/assessments in practice I am not getting the support I would like to have
RED *	I am dissatisfied with the direction of my life I feel, I am not able to handle things anymore I am getting irritated and stressed out in placement, in university and at home I am having negative thoughts and feeling petrified about going to lectures and on placement I am not getting support from anyone in the university, on placement or from family and friends

Table 10.2   Assessing My Social Health: Abesola

Who am I connecting with in my home?	Make a list or if you are feeling creative draw the people who you are connecting with
Who am I connecting with whilst I am completing my modules/my programme of study in university?	Make a list or if you are feeling creative draw the people who you are connecting with
Who am I connecting with when I am in clinical practice?	Make a list or if you are feeling creative draw the people who you are connecting with
Who am I connecting with whilst working on my assignments?	Make a list Or if you are feeling creative draw the people who you are connecting with
Who am I connecting with as my assignment/exam deadlines are pending?	Make a list Or if you are feeling creative draw the people who you are connecting with
Who am I connecting with to get support?	Make a list or if you are feeling creative draw the people who you are connecting with

Table 10.3   Interpreting my social health

Green ****	I am in regular contact with family and friends I meet up with colleagues students on the course regularly I organise to meet my PT/lecturers when I am at university I meet with practice supervisor/assessor weekly to have an update on my progress I go home and spend time with family and friends I have evenings out with my friends
Amber ***	I tend to retreat from meeting people I don't have many connections with other students I don't tend to meet with colleagues in clinical practice till I am requested to do so I don't bother to see my personal tutor and lecturers I emotionally distant from family and important people in my life

(Continued)

Table 10.3 Interpreting my social health *(Continued)*

RED **	I do not want to engage with fellow students in the university or colleagues in clinical practice I am not keeping in touch with family and friends I feel fearful of connecting with people I dread engaging in social activities with anyone

Table 10.4 Assessing My Financial Health: Abesola

What are my sources of income this month?

What is my total income this month?

How much have I spent this month?

Am I in credit or deficit? if so by how much?

I am in credit. What is my credit?

Can I use my credit I have?

I am in deficit. What is my deficit?

Will I be able to clear my deficit soon, if so, how?

Do I need financial advice and support and where can I find help?

Table 10.5 Interpreting my financial health

GREEN ***	I am in credit at the end of the month I am able to afford to spend on special occasions I feel confident about how to manage my income effectively I can access extra income if necessary I feel confident that if I need to budget, I will be able to do so
AMBER **	I am in debt some months and then it's not easy to stay in credit I work with a tight budget and not always able to save for special occasions Sometimes, I can really make savings when I try I do know where to get financial help if I need it Generally, I am more in debt than in credit
RED *	I am in debt every month I never seem able to keep to within my spending budget I make big spends regularly even though I don't have the money I keep borrowing more money and now in serious debt I owe a lot of money to a lot of people

What are the results of the self-assessment of my physical, psychological, social and financial health?

Put my findings/results on a chart: Abesola (Table 10.6)

Table 10.6 My self-assessment results/findings: Abesola

Results	Green or ****	Amber or ***	Red or **
Physical health		Amber or ***	
Psychological health			Red or **
Social health		Amber or ***	
Financial health			Red **

What does these results mean for me? Asebola (Table 10.7)

Table 10.7 What does my self-assessment results mean?

Physical Health	AMBER ***
Exercise	I exercise 2-3 times a week
Rest and relaxation	I do get some rest each week, but I don't meditate/ undertake any relaxation
Eating	I eat on time generally and I do have some healthy but mostly I have meats fried and sweet foods
Hydration	I drink when I remember to do so. I do prefer coffee/tea mostly
Sleep	I get good sleep some nights but I toss and turn a lot. Generally, I get about 5-6 hours sleep each
Alcohol intake	I have 2-3 large glasses of wine or 2 pints of larger daily
Blood pressure and BMI	My BP is 130/90 and My BMI 25
Psychological Health	**RED ****
	I am dissatisfied with the direction of my life
	I feel, I am not able to handle things anymore
	I am getting irritated and stressed out in placement, in university and at home
	I am having negative thoughts and feeling petrified about going to lectures and on placement
	I am not getting support from anyone in the university, on placement or from family and friends

(Continued)

Table 10.7　What does my self-assessment results mean? *(Continued)*

Social Health	Amber ***
	I tend to retreat from meeting people
	I don't have many connections with other students
	I don't tend to meet with colleagues in clinical practice till I am requested to do so
	I don't bother to see my personal tutor and lecturers
	I am emotionally distant from family and the important people in my life
Financial Health	**RED ****
	I am in debt every month
	I never seem able to keep to within my spending budget
	I make big spends regularly even though I don't have the money
	I keep borrowing more money and now in serious debt
	I owe a lot of money to a lot of people

These are my personal goals and actions to achieve a higher level of personal wellbeing: Asebola

Physical health

- Increase my daily exercise
- Increase my rest time
- Introduce a healthy programme of eating
- Drink more water daily
- Improve my sleeping to 7–8 hours nightly
- Limit my wine intake
- Lower my BP
- Lower my BMI

Psychological health: Feeling and Thoughts

- Reduce my level of stress
- Introduce positive thought
- Reduce my anxiety levels
- Find my coping strategies

Social health

- Improve my social contacts
- Expand my connections
- Connect with my family and key people in my life

Financial health

- Improve my financial situation
- Reduce my spending
- Clear my debt as soon as possible
- Seek financial help

Asebola's goals and actions

1 **Physical Health**
   Goal: Increase my daily exercise
   Actions

- Take a daily walk in the local park on my days off
- Daily walks to university or placement – perhaps come off one bus or train stop earlier and walk
- Join a gym
- Join a local exercise class
- Daily walk with a friend
- Join a local walking group

Goal: Increase my rest time
Actions
- Set aside time to rest daily
- Have a power nap when I can
- Do mindfulness/yoga/meditation daily

Goal: Introduce my healthy programme of eating
Actions
Start off by cutting down on
- fried foods
- processed foods
- fizzy drinks
- cakes and chocolates

Eat more
- oily fish
- legume and beans
- vegetables
- fruits
- chicken
- have a dollop of natural yorgurt daily on its own
- drink plenty of water

Goal: Drink more water daily
Actions

- Buy a plastic recycle bottle
- Drink water at every opportunity
- Increase tea intake

Goal: Improve my sleeping to 7–8 hours nightly
Actions

- Think and see bedroom as a place of rest, sleep and relaxation
- Avoid social media activity well before bed
- Drink a relaxing drink
- Make sure pillows are comfortable
- Read/listen to relaxing music

Goal: Limit my wine intake
Actions

- Assess whether drinking is social
- Set a limit during social activity
- Try non-alcoholic drinks
- Seek support to help you if you feel you need it

Goal: Lower my BP and lower my BMI
Actions

- Increase exercise
- Increase relaxation
- Change your diet, go for healthy options
- Join an activity group
- Contact my GP to check my BP often

2 **Psychological Health: Can you identify what actions Asebola needs to set to improve her Psychological Health?**
   Goal: Reduce my level of stress
   Actions

   Goal: Reduce my anxieties
   Actions

   Goal: Develop positive thoughts and feelings
   Actions

   Goal: Develop coping strategies
   Actions

3 **Social health**
    Goal: Improve my social contacts
    Actions

- Join a local group – walking/dancing/reading
- Start a new class
- Join a community group
- Join a cultural group
- Join student union
- Talk to student union

    Goal: Expand my connections
    Actions

- Talk to peers in your lecturers
- Contact your personal tutor
- Join in cultural activities
- Go to student café/canteen and sit with peers
- Set up your own social group

    Goal: Connect with family and key people in her life
    Actions

- Reach out to family and friend who you have not connected with recently by phone, WhatsApp, email or letter
- Organise a family catch up
- Meet up for a coffee
- Meet at church or at a cultural activity
- Meet for a walk and talk

4 **Financial Health: Can you identify what actions Asebola needs to take to improve her Financial Health?**
    Goal: Improve my financial situation
    Actions

    Goal: Reduce spending
    Actions

    Goal: Clear my debt
    Actions

Personal Wellbeing Diary: Set Your Daily Goals

Table 10.8 Personal wellbeing diary: Set you daily goals

Monday	Tuesday	Wednesday	Thursday	Friday	Saturday	Sunday

Tips for Self-Motivation

1 Action for Happiness

Create your own daily happiness calendar (many online) Write in daily thoughts/actions/activity or access one from the site below that already has daily activities/actions/thoughts

https://actionforhappiness.org/all-calendars

Your own action for happiness calendar: Example (Table 10.9)

Table 10.9 My happiness calendar

Monday	Tuesday	Wednesday	Thursday	Friday	Saturday	Sunday
Change my mood by doing something different	Write down all the positive things in my life					

2 My own gratitude journal (Figure 10.3)

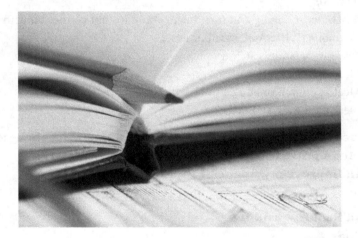

Figure 10.3 Gratitude journal

Reviewing My Progress: Write Down Your Weekly Progress Towards Achieving Your Goals and Actions

Table 10.10 Review of my progress

Week 1
Week 2
Week 3
Week 4
Week 5
Week 6

Reset Your Plans

Once you have reviewed your goals and action, if you need to reset your goals, you can use the same resources used for goal planning above.

Resources for Your Use

NHS-BMI calculator

https://www.nhs.uk/conditions/obesity/
Blood Pressure check: See your GP for a health check

Health eating

https://www.nhs.uk/live-well/eat-well/how-to-eat-a-balanced-diet/eight-tips-for-healthy-eating/

Eating for healthy heart BHF

https://www.bhf.org.uk/informationsupport/support/healthy-living/healthy-eating

Alcohol support

https://www.nhs.uk/live-well/alcohol-advice/alcohol-support/

Smoking support

https://www.nhs.uk/better-health/quit-smoking/

NHS Mental health tools and activities

- Wellbeing self-assessment
- Mood self-assessment
- Depression self-assessment
- Mental health video wall
- Lift your mood video wall

   https://www.nhs.uk/mental-health/self-help/guides-tools-and-activities/depression-anxiety-self-assessment-quiz/

NHS Employers Assessment Tools/activities

https://www.nhsemployers.org/howareyoufeelingnhs

NHS wellbeing tool kit

https://www.nhsemployers.org/howareyoufeelingnhs
    https://www.england.nhs.uk/supporting-our-nhs-people/support-now/well-being-apps/

NHS approved apps

A list of NHS approved apps and online tools to help you manage and improve your health

Apps and Podcasts

Headspace

Headspace is a mobile app which makes practicing mindfulness much easier! Helping you learn easy techniques that you can transfer from the session into your everyday life. You can sign up for free on their **Take 10** programme – *just 10 minutes a day for 10 days.*

Breathe

Breathe is a mindfulness app that helps you stay calm and battle anxiety by sending you gentle deep breathing reminders throughout the day.

Mental Health Foundation

Have a look at this link to download free wellbeing podcasts on mindfulness, exercise, diet, relaxation, stress and anxiety.

Emoodji

Emoodji is an app created by Mind, designed specifically for students. Uni life can have its ups and downs, but Emoodji is there throughout. It is a fun way of looking after yourself, sharing with friends and supporting each other.

Happify

An app aimed at developing skills in order to boost emotional wellbeing.

Useful Websites

Student Minds

Student Minds is the United Kingdom's student mental health charity. Their website features lots of really useful resources on a variety of topics, including:

- Starting university
- Looking after your mental wellbeing
- Exam stress
- Year abroad
- LGBTQ+
- Student Finance
- University life through a family health crisis

Blurt

Mental health toolkit, self-care starter kit, a list of more useful apps and more.

Mental Health Foundation

The Mental Health Foundation offers a range of information to inform and encourage a greater understanding of how to look after your mental health, as well as an A–Z guide of mental health

https://www.nih.gov/health-information/social-wellness-toolkit

https://www.england.nhs.uk/supporting-our-nhs-people/health-and-wellbeing-programmes/nhs-health-and-wellbeing-framework/elements-of-health-and-wellbeing/improving-personal-health-and-wellbeing/

Chapter Summary

In this final chapter, we have provided you with some tips to help you bring about personal change in order to improve and maintain your wellbeing. We demonstrated how to set out, implement and monitor your own personal wellbeing and how to create your own journal. We created an assessment tools which we used to assess physical, psychological, social and financial health of an individual. We then used the evidence from the assessment of the individuals' holistic health to set out personal goals and action. We have created an example to illustrate how you can go about setting your goals and steps to achieve your goals. Once you have implemented your action plans, we suggest you review it regularly and create a tool to do so. We realise that change is not easy and so we have given you some tips to keep you self-motivated. We have given you access to a range of resources to help improve and maintain your wellbeing whilst on your studies and beyond. Your personal wellbeing is essential not only to yourself and your family but to the profession you are joining and the patients, service users and clients in your care.

References

Aaslund, H. (2021). Global experiences of social work practice during the pandemic: Digital mediums, mutual aid, and professional self-care. *Qualitative Social Work*, 20(1–2), 375–377.

Aiken, L., Servmous, W., Vanden Heede, K., Sloane, D., Busse, R., Mckee, M., Bruyneel, L., Rafferty, A., Griffiths, P., Moreno-Casbas, T., Tishelman, C., Scott, P., Brzostek, T., Kinnunen, J., Schwendimann, R., Heinen, M., Zikos, D., Sjetne, I., Smith, H., & Kutney-Lee, A. (2012). Patient safety, satisfaction, and quality of hospital care: Cross sectional surveys of nurses and patients in 12 countries in Europe and the United States. *British Medical Journal*, 344, e1717. https://doi.org/10.1136/bmj.e1717

All-Party Parliamentary Group on Arts, Health and Wellbeing (APPGAHW). (2017). In *Creative health: The arts for health and wellbeing*. Inquiry Report (2nd ed.). http://www.artshealthandwellbeing.org.uk/appg-inquiry/

Allen, S. (2018). *The science of gratitude. A white book*. John Templeton Foundation. https://ggsc.berkeley.edu/images/uploads/GGSC-JTF_White_Paper-Gratitude-FINAL.pdf

Apostolidou, C., Adamopoulos, K., Lymperaki, E., Iliadis, S., Papapreponis, P., & Kourtidou-Papadeli, C. (2015). Cardiovascular risk and benefits from antioxidant dietary intervention with red wine in asymptomatic hypercholesterolemics. *Clinical Nutrition ESPEN*, 10(6), e224–e233.

Arimitsu, K., & Stefan, G. H. (2015). Effect of compassionate thinking on negative emotion. *Cognition and Emotion*, 31(1), 160–167. https://doi.org/10.1080/02699931.2015.1078292

Atkinson, K., Edginton, T., & Noble, H. (2021). Mindfullness as a well-being initiative for future nurses: A survey with undergraduate nursing students. *BMC Nursing*, 20(253), 1–9.

Ball, J., Maben, J., Murrells, T., Day, T., & Griffiths, P. (2014). *12-hour shifts: Prevalence, views and impact*. National Nursing Research Unit, King's College London. NHS England Publications Gateway Reference: 03620.

Barrett, L. F. (2018). In *How emotions are made: The secret life of the Brain* (2nd ed.). Pan Books.

BBC. (2019). *Even a small amount of creativity can help you cope with modern life, reveals new research by BBC Arts and UCL*. https://www.bbc.co.uk/mediacentre/latestnews/2019/get-creative-research

Bond, M., Buntins, K., Bedenlier, S., Zawacki- Richter, O., & Kerres, M. (2020). Mapping research in student engagement and educational technology in higher education: A systematic evidence map. *International Journal of Educational Technology in Higher Education*, 17(2). https://doi.org/10.1186/s41239-019-0176-8

Brockman, R., Ciarrochi, J., Parker, P., & Kashdan, T. (2016). Emotion regulation strategies in daily life: Mindfulness, cognitive reappraisal and emotion suppression. *Cognitive Behavioral Therapy*, 46(2), 91–113. https://doi.org/10.1080/16506073.2016.1218926

Bryson, C. (2014). *Understanding and developing student engagement*. London: Routledge.

Buckley, A. (2014). How radical is student engagement? (and what is it for?). *Student Engagement and Experience Journal*, 3(2), 1–23. https://doi.org/10.7190/seej.v3i2.95

Butler and Hope. (1995). *The worry tree*. https://positivepsychology.com/mental-health-exercises-interventions/

Carless, D. (2015). *Excellence in university assessment: Learning from award-winning teaching*. Routledge.

Cherry, K. (2020). *The 6 types of basic emotions and their effect on human behaviour*. Very Well Mind. The 6 Types of Basic Emotions. verywellmind.com

Codier, E. (2020). *Emotional intelligence in nursing: Essentials for leadership and practice improvement*. Springer.

Colin, B. (2014). *Understanding and developing student engagement*. Routledge. https://doi.org/10.4324/9781315813691

Cottrell, S. (2018). *Mindfulness for students* (1st ed.). Palgrave.

Cottrell, S. (2019). In *The study skills handbook* (5th ed.). Red Globe Press and Macmillan.

Cowen, A. S., & Keltner, D. (2017). Self report captures 27 distinct categories of emotion bridged by continuous gradients. *Psychological and Cognitive Sciences*, 114(38), 7900–7909.

Craig, A., Hansen, R. J., Knopf, R. C., Thaxton, S. P., McTague, R., & Bennett Moore, D. (2019). The unleashing the value of lifelong learning institutes: Research and practice insights from a national survey of Osher lifelong learning institutes. *Adult Education Quarterly*, 69(3), 184–206.

Damasio, A. (2018). *Strange order of things: Life, feeling and the making of cultures*. Pantheon Books.

Damasio, A. (2021). *Feeling and knowing: Making minds conscious*. Robinson.

Dahlgren, G., & Whitehead, M. (1991). *Policies and strategies to promote social equity in health*. Stockholm: Institute for Futures Studies.

David, S. (2016). *3 Ways to better understand your emotions*. Harvard Business Review. https://hbr.org/2016/11/3-ways-to-better-understand-your-emotions

De Hert, S. (2020). Burnout in healthcare workers: Prevalence, impact and preventative strategies. *Local and Regional Anesthesia*, 13, 171–183. https://doi.org/10.2147/LRA.S240564

Department of Health. (2012). *Health and social care act*. HMSO.

Department of Health. (2014). *Five year forward view*. HMSO.

Department of Health and Social Care. (2021). *Guidance the NHS constitution for England*. https://www.gov.uk/government/publications/the-nhs-constitution-for-england/the-nhs-constitution-for-england

Diener, E., Pressman, S. D., Hunter, J., & Delgadillo-Chase, D. (2017). If, why, and when subjective well-being influences health, and future needed research. *Applied Psychology: Health and Well-Being*, 9(2), 133–167. https://doi.org/10.1111/aphw. 12090. PMID: 28707767.

Edwards, N. (2010). There's so much potential...and for whatever reason it's not being realized – women's relationships with midwives as a negotiation of ideology and practice. In M. Kirkham (Ed.), *The midwife-mother relationship*. Palgrave, Macmillan.

Ekman, P. (1984). Expression and the nature of emotion. In K. Scherer & P. Ekman (Eds.), *Approaches to emotion*. Erlbaum.

Ekman, P. (1992). An argument for basic emotions. *Cognition & Emotion*, 6(3–4), 169–200.

Ekman, P. (1999). Basic emotions. *Handbook of Cognition and Emotion*, 98(45–60), 16.

Elcock, K. (2020). *How to succeed on nursing placements*. SAGE Publications.

Engel, G. (1977). The need for a new medical model: A challenge for biomedicine. *Science*, 196(4286), 129–136.

Fasbinder, A., Shidler, K., & Caboral-Stevens, M. (2020). A concept analysis: Emotional regulation for nurses. *Nursing Forum*, 55, 118–127.

Gemine, R., Davies, G. R., Tarrant, S., Davies, R. M., James, M., & Lewis, K. (2021). Factors associated with work-related burnout in NHS staff during COVID-19: A cross-sectional mixed methods study. *BMJ Open*, 11(1), e042591. https://doi.org/10.1136/bmjopen-2020-042591

Ghisoni, M., & Murphy, P. (2019). *Study skills: For nursing, health and social care*. Lantern Publishing.

Goleman, D. (1995). *Emotional intelligence: Why it can matter more than IQ*. Bantam Books.

Goleman, D. (1998). *Working with emotional intelligence*. Bloomsbury.

Gov.uk. (2017). *Future of skills and lifelong learning*. publishing.service.gov.uk

Gross, J. J. (2015). Emotional regulation: Current status and future prospects. *Psychological Inquiry*, 26, 1–26. https://doi-org.ezproxy.uwl.ac.uk/10.1080/1047 840X.201

Hagemeister, A., & Volmer, J. (2018). Developing emotional regulation skills in the workplace. *Human Resource Management International Digest*, 26(4), 19–21.

Hallam, K. T., Bilsborough, S., & de Courten, M. (2018). "Happy feet": Evaluating the benefits of A 100-day 10,000 step challenge on mental health and wellbeing. *BMC Psychiatry*, 18(19), 1–7.

Hazard, L., & Carter, S. (2018). A framework for helping families understand the college transition. *E-source for College Transitions*, 16(1), 13–15.

Health & Care Professional Council hcpc. (2018). *Standards of education and training. Standards of proficiency*. https://www.hcpc-uk.org/education/resources/education-standards/

Health and Safety Executive. (2017). *Tackling work-related stress using the management standards approach*. https://www.hse.gov.uk/pubns/wbk01.pdf

Holloway, S., Taylor, A., & Tombs, M. (2020). Impact of postgraduate study on healthcare professionals' academic and clinical practice. *British Journal of Healthcare Management*, 26(7). https://doi-org.ezproxy.uwl.ac.uk/10.12968/bjhc.2019.0058

Hone, L. (2017). *Resilence grieving; How to find way through a devastating loss. Finding strength and embracing life after a loss that changes everything.* Allen & Urwin.

Huffington, A. (2014). *Thrive.* Penguin Random House.

Hunter, B. (2004). Conflicting ideologies as a source of emotion work in midwifery. *Midwifery,* 20(3), 261–272. https://doi.org/10.1016/j.midw.2003.12.004

Hunter, B. (2009). Mixed messages: Midwives' experiences of managing emotion. In B. Hunter & R. Deery (Eds.), *Emotions in midwifery and reproduction.* Palgrave Macmillan.

Hunter, B. (2010). Mapping the emotional terrain of midwifery: What can we see and what lies ahead? *International Journal of Work Organisation and Emotion,* 3(3), 253–269.

Juckel, G., Heinisch, C., Welpinghus, A., & Brüne, M. (2018). Understanding another person's emotions-an interdisciplinary research approach. *Frontiers in Psychiatry,* 9, 414. https://doi.org/10.3389/fpsyt.2018.00414

Kayral, I., & Dülger, D. (2019). The impact of self-leadership skills of healthcare employees on institutional performance and job performance. *Journal of Basic and Clinical Health Sciences,* 3, 145–150.

Kelly, N. J., Glazer, J. E., Porpattananangkul, N., & Nusslock, R. (2018). Reappraisal and suppression emotion – regulation tendencies differentially predict reward-responsivity ad psychological well-being. *Biological Psychology,* 140, 35–47.

King's Fund. (2018). *The healthcare workforce in England: Make or break?* https://www.kingsfund.org.uk/publications/health-care-workforce-england

Kings Fund. (2019). *Community health services explained.* Kings Fund. https://www.kingsfund.org.uk/publications/community-health-services-explained

Kirk, K., Cohen, L., Egley, A., & Timmons, S. (2021). "I don't have any emotions" an ethnography of emotional labour and feeling rules in the emergency department, *Journal of Advanced Nursing,* 77(4), 1956–1967.

Koch, C. (2018). What is consciousness?. *Nature,* 557, S8–S12. https://doi.org/10.1038/d41586-018-05097-x

Kotsou, I., Mikolajczak, M., Heeren, A., Grégoire, J., & Leys, C. (2019). Improving emotional intelligence: A systematic review of existing work and future challenges. *Emotion Review,* 11(2), 151–165. https://doi.org/10.1177/1754073917735902

Lauren, T., Gandhi, J., & Sharma, S. (2022). https://cdn.locals.com/documents/285938/285938_9w4pjridyepu95c.pdf

Linsley, P. (2011). In P. Linsley, R. Kane & S. Owen (Eds.), *Nursing for public health* (1st ed.). University Press.

MacDonald, M. (2018). *Training nurses, midwives and nursing associates: The student voice.* https://www.nmc.org.uk/globalassets/sitedocuments/education-standards/the-student-voice-v2.pdf

Manstead, T. (2005). The social dimension of emotion. *The Psychologist,* 18(8), 184–187.

Manz, C. C. (1983). Improving performance through self-leadership. *National Productivity Review,* 2(3), 288–297.

Maye, J. G., & Geher, G. (1996). Emotional intelligence and the identification of emotion. *Intelligence,* 22(2), 89–113. https://doi.org/10.1016/s0160-2896(96)90011-2

Mayer, J. D., Caruso, D. R., & Salovey, P. (1999). Emotional intelligence meets traditional standards for an intelligence. *Intelligence*, 27(4), 267–298. https://doi.org/10.1016/S0160-2896(99)00016-1

McGrath, L., Swift, A., Clark, M., & Bradley-Jones, C. (2019). Understanding the benefits and risks of nursing students engaging with online social media. *Nursing Standard*, 34(10), 45–49. https://doi.org/10.7748/ns.2019.e11362

McVeigh, C., Reid, J., Carswell, C., Ace, L., Walsh, I., Graham-Wisener, L., Rej, S. P., & McGonigal, K. (2021). *The upside of stress: Why stress is good for you and how to get good at it.* Vermilion.

Mills, A., Ryden, J., & Knight, A. (2020). Juggling to find balance: Hearing the voices of undergraduate student nurses. *British Journal of Nursing*, 29(4), 897–903.

Mitchell, A. (2022). *Supporting the failing student week 7.* Milton Keynes: Open University (OU).

Nagoski, E., & Nagoski, A. (2020). In *Burnout: Solve your stress cycle* (2nd ed.). Vermillion.

National Health Service (NHS) England. (2014). *Building and strengthening leadership leading with compassion.* NHS England. https://www.england.nhs.uk/wp-content/uploads/2014/12/london-nursing-accessible.pdf

National Health Service (NHS) England. (2018). *NHS staff survey available*: National NHS Staff Survey 2018 – GOV.UK. www.gov.uk

Nehrlich, A. D., Gebauer, J. E., Sedikides, C., & Abele, A. E. (2019). Individual self relational self collective self-but why? Processes driving the self-hierarchy in self- and person perception. *Journal of Personality*, 8(2), 212–230.

NHS Digital. (2021). NHS sickness absence rates July 2020 to September 2020, provisional statistics In: *NHS sickness absence rates.* https://digital.nhs.uk/data-and-information/publications/statistical/nhs-sickness-absence-rates/july-2020-to-september-2020-provisional-statistics

NHS Employers. (2021). *Supporting our NHS people experiencing stress.* https://www.nhsemployers.org/articles/supporting-our-nhs-people-experiencing-stress

NHS England. (2017). *A-EQUIP a model of clinical midwifery supervision.* https://www.england.nhs.uk/publication/a-equip-a-model-of-clinical-midwifery-supervision/

NHS England. (2019). *NHS staff survey.* https://www.nhsstaffsurveys.com/

NHS England. (2021). *Professional nurse advocate A-EQUIP model: A model of clinical supervision for nurses.* https://www.england.nhs.uk/publication/professional-nurse-advocate-a-equip-model-a-model-of-clinical-supervision-for-nurses/

NHS England. (2022). *Primary care services.* NHS England. https://www.england.nhs.uk/get-involved/get-involved/how/primarycare/

Nursing and Midwifery Council NMC. (2018). *Future nurses: Standard of proficiency for registered nurses.* https://www.nmc.org.uk/globalassets/sitedocuments/standards/nmc-standards-of-proficiency-for-preregistration-nursing-education.pdf

ONS (Office for National Statistics). (2021). *Personal wellbeing in the UK: April 2020–March 2021.* https://www.ons.gov.uk/peoplepopulationandcommunity/wellbeing/bulletins/measuringnationalwellbeing/april2020tomarch2021

Parra, L. A., Bell, T. S., Benibgui, M., Helm, J. L., & Hastings, P. D. (2018). The buffering effect of peer support on the links between family rejection and psychosocial adjustment in LGB emerging adults. *Journal of Social and Personal Relationships*, 35(6), 854–871.

Partridge, C. (2020). *Wake up: What your emotions are trying to tell you*. 3-Heads Publishing.

Pena-Sarrionandia, A., Mikolajcak, M., & Gross, J. (2015). Integrating emotional regulation and emotional intelligence traditions: A meta-analysis. *Frontiers in Psychology*, 6(160), 22–26.

Quick, J. C., & Spielberger, C. D. (1994). Walter Bradford Cannon: Pioneer of stress research. *International Journal of Stress Manage*, 1, 141–143. https://doi.org/10.1007/BF01857607

Ragau, S., Hitchcock, R., Craft, J., & Christensen, M. (2018). Using the HALT model in an exploratory quality improvement initiative to reduce medication errors. *The British Journal of Nursing*, 27(22), 1330–1335. https://doi.org/10.12968/bjon.2018.27.22.1330. PMID: 30525975.

Ramage, C., & Moorley, C. (2019). A narrative synthesis on healthcare students use and understanding of social media: Implications for practice. *Nurse Education Today*, 77, 40–52. https://doi.org/10.1016/j.nedt.2019.03.010

Ramscar, M., Hendrix, P., Shaoul, C., Milin, P., & Baayen, H. (2014). The myth of cognitive decline: Non-linear dynamics of lifelong learning. *Topics in Cognitive Science*, 6, 5–42. https://doi-org.ezproxy.uwl.ac.uk/10.111/tops.12078

Rangel, A. (2018). A test of the main-effects, stress-buffering, stress-exacerbation, and joint-effects models among Mexican-origin adults. *Journal of Latina/o Psychology*, 7(3), 212–229.

RCN. (2022). *Working time and breaks*. https://www.rcn.org.uk/get-help/rcn-advice/working-time-rest-breaks-on-call-and-night-work

Reamer, F. G. (2013). Social work in a digital age: Ethical and risk management challenges. *Social Work*, 58(2), 163–172. http://www.jstor.org/stable/23719783

Rodriguez, N., Flores, R. T., London, E. F., Bingham, M. C., Myers, H. F., Arroyo, D., & Rimmer, A. (2018). Staff stress levels reflect rising pressure on NHS, says NHS leaders. *British Medical Journal*, 360, k1074. https://doi.org/10.1136/bmj.k1074

Rogers, R., Neve, A., Rees, H., Tomlinson, A., & Williams, G. (2020). COVID-19 and student nurses: A view from England. *Journal of Clinical Nursing*, 29, 3111–3114. https://doi.org/10.1111/jocn.15298

Royal College Nursing. (2021). *Healthy workplace toolkit*. https://www.rcn.org.uk/professional-development/publications/healthy-workplace-toolkit-uk-pub-009-734

Ruggeri, K., Garcia-Garzon, E., Maguire, Á., Matz, S., & Huppert, F. (2020). Well-being is more than happiness and life satisfaction: A multidimensional analysis of 21 countries. *Health and Quality of Life Outcomes*, 18, 192. https://doi.org/10.1186/s12955-020-01423-y

Ruotsalainen, J. H., Verbeek, J. H., Mariné, A., & Serra, C. (2015). Preventing occupational stress in healthcare workers. *The Cochrane Database of Systematic Reviews*, 2015(4), CD002892. https://doi.org/10.1002/14651858.CD002892.pub5

Salovey, P., & Mayer, J. D. (1990). Emotional intelligence. *Imagination, Cognition, and Personality*, 9, 185–211.

Satpute, A. B., Nook, E. C., Narayanan, S., Shu, J., Weber, J., & Ochsner, K. N. (2016). Emotions in "black and white" or shades of gray? How we think about emotions shapes our perception and neural representation of emotion. *Association for Psychological Science*, 27(11), 1428–1442. https://doi.org/10.1177/0956797616661555

Sermeus, W., Aiken, K., Van den Heede, A., Marie Rafferty, A., Griffiths, P., Teresa Moreno-Casbas, M., Busse, R., Lindqvist, R., Scott, A. P., Bruyneel, L., Brzostek, T., Kinnunen, J., Schubert, M., Schoonhoven, L., & Zikos, D. (2011). Nurse forecasting in Europe (RN4CAST): Rationale, design and methodology. *BMC Nursing*, 10, 6.

Serrat, O. (2017). Understanding and developing emotional intelligence. In: *Knowledge solutions*. Springer. https://doi.org/10.1007/978-981-10-0983-9_37

Shi, M., Jiang, R., Hu, X., & Shang, J. (2019). A privacy protection method for health care big data management based on risk access control. *Health Care Management Science*, 23, 427–442. https://doi.org/10.1007/s10729-019-09490-4

Short, E. (2021). *A prescription for healthy living: A guide to lifestyle medicine*. Academic Press.

Siegel, D. J. (2020). In *The developing mind: How relationships and the brain interact to shape who we are* (3rd ed.). The Guilford Press.

Skinner, E. A., & Belmont, M. J. (1993). Motivation in the classroom: Reciprocal effects of teacher behavior and student engagement across the school year. *Journal of Educational Psychology*, 85(4), 571–581. https://doi.org/10.1037/0022-0663.85.4.571

Smith, P. (2012). In *The emotional labour of nursing revisited: Can nurses still care?* (2nd ed.). Palgrave MacMillan.

Smith, J. A.; Newman, K. M.; Suttie, J., & Jazaieri, H. (2017). The state of mindfulness science. *Greater Good Magazine*. https://greatergood.berkeley.edu/article/item/the_state_of_mindfulness_science

Social Work England. (2019). *Education and training standards*. SWE. https://www.socialworkengland.org.uk/standards/education-and-training-standards/

Solaas, S. A., & Kleppang, A. L. (2022). Association between physical activity, sedentary time, participation in organized activities, social support, sleep problems and mental distress among adults in Southern Norway: A cross-sectional study among 28,047 adults from the general population. *BMC Public Health*, 22(384), 1–11.

Stamatakis, E. (2013). Is the lack of physical activity strategy for children complicit mass child neglect. *British Medical Journal*, 48(13), 1010–1013. Stea

Swift, A., Banks, L., Baleswaran, A., Cooke, N., Little, C., McGrath, L., & Meechan-Rogers, R. (2020). COVID-19 and student nurses: A view from England. *Journal of Clinical Nursing*, 29(17–18), 3111–3114.

Swift, A., & Twycross, A. (2020). The challenges of being a student nurse and the advice proffered by peers. *Evidence-Based Nursing*, 23(1), 8–10.

Tantam, D. (2014). *Emotional wellbeing and mental health: A guide for counsellors and psychotherapists*. SAGE.

The British Association of Social Workers (2018). *Social media Policy*. https://www.basw.co.uk/resources/basws-social-media-policy

Thomas, R. (2021). In *How to promote wellbeing: Practical steps for healthcare practitioner's mental health* (1st ed.). Wiley Blackwell.

Thomas, P. A., Liu, H., & Umberson, D. (2017). Family relationships and well-being. *Innovation in Aging*, 1(3). https://doi.org/10.1093/geroni/igx025

Traynor, M. (2017). *Critical resilience for nursing*. Routledge.

UNESCO Institute for Lifelong Learning. (2022). *Lifelong learning opportunities for all: Medium-term strategy 2022–2029*. UNESCO Institute for Lifelong Learning. https://unesdoc.unesco.org/ark:/48223/pf0000380778

Upton, K. V. (2018). An investigation into compassion fatigue and self-compassion in acute medical care hospital nurses: A mixed methods study. *Journal of Compassionate Health Care*, 5(1), 7.

van Dorssen-Boog, P., de Jong, J., Veld, M., & Van Vuuren, T. (2020). Self-leadership among healthcare workers: A mediator for the effects of job autonomy on work engagement and health. *Frontiers in Psychology*, 11, 1420.

Veigh, C. M., Reid, J., Carswell, C., Ace, L., Walsh, I., Graham-Wisener, L., & Rej, S. (2021). Mindfulness as a well-being initiative for future nurses: A survey with undergraduate nursing students. *BMC Nursing*, 20, 253. https://doi.org/10.1186/s12912-021-00783-0

Webb, L. (2013). *Resilence: How to cope when everything around you keeps changing*. Capstone.

West, M. S., & Chowla, R. (2017). Compassionate leadership for compassionate health care. In P. Gilbert (Ed.), *Compassion: Concepts, research and applications* (pp. 237–257). Routledge.

West, M., Collins, B., Eckert, R., & Chowla, R. (2017). *Caring to change: How compassionate leadership can stimulate innovation in health care*. https://www.kingsfund.org.uk/publications/caring-change

World Health Organization. (2020). Health and wellbeing. https://www.who.int/data/gho/data/major-themes/health-and-well-being

World Health Organization. (2019). *The WHO special initiative for mental health (2019–2023): Universal health coverage for mental health*. World Health Organization.

Wright, N., Zakarian, M., & Blake, H. (2016). Nurses views on workplace wellbeing programmes. *British Journal of Nursing*, 25(21), 1208–1212.

Zych, A. D., & Gogolla, N. (2021). Expressions of emotions across species. *Science Direct Elsevier*, 68, 57–66.

Annotated list of useful websites

Building lifelong skills for lifelong learning in the 21st century: How to build lifelong learning skills for the 21st century workplace (cambridgeassessment.org.uk)

- How to create a learning plan How to Create a Personal Learning Plan – From MindTools.com
- 10 things to do before starting your university course 10 things to do before starting university | Prospects.ac.uk
- What is life really like as a paramedic student? 5 Things I Wish I Knew Before Becoming A Student Paramedic (healthjobs.co.uk)

- What is life really like at university? Listen to student stories and get some useful tips What university is really like | The Student Room
- Life as a paramedic Information on being a paramedic – Degrees and Courses – NHS Careers (healthcareers.nhs.uk)
- Top tips for young students going to university – Tips for Young Students at College or University – YouTube
- It is never too late to learn – Oldest school students show it's never too late to learn – Theirworld
- Academic integrity. https://www.rlf.org.uk/resources/mla-apa-harvard-or-mhra/ #:~:text=Referencing%20styles,Modern%20Humanities%20Research%20Associ ation)%20system.
- Emotional adjustment
  180531_transitions_interactive.pdf (studentminds.org.uk)
  What to do when you feel homesick | Prospects.ac.uk
  3 Tips to help International Students Adjust to a New Country (edaptapp.com)
- Financial
  Financial support for students not supported by their parents (estranged) | Undergraduate, Conservatoires | UCAS
  8 Tips on How to Adjust to University Life – AHZ Associates
  Money and budgeting | British Council
  https://www.ucas.com/undergraduate/applying-university/individual-needs/students-parenting-responsibilities -
  https://www.whatuni.com/advice/guides/ultimate-guide-to-student-volunteering/76054/
  Social media usage in the United Kingdom (UK) – statistics & facts | Statista
- The University of California, Los Angeles (UCLA) Mindful Awareness Research Centre (MARC) has a free, comprehensive and simple app with different mindful related resources available so you can focus on your wellbeing. From self-learning meditation to informative podcasts, the UCLA Mindful App is available for iOS and Android users.
- Prospect the University of Oxford Mindfulness Centre and find free online podcasts and practice sessions https://www.oxfordmindfulness.org/
- The Fitmind podcasts, founded by Liam McClintock, brings different experts' contributions in different healthy mind-related areas. You can access all of its podcasts contributions here: https://www.fitmind.co/podcast and specific playlists such as creating healthy mind on their YouTube channel: https:// www.youtube.com/channel/UC8_eJSJPnsMlfk0Sr4DreNA
- Visit the Greater Good Science Centre at University of California, Berkeley (UC Berkeley) website where you can find podcasts by topic, keys to wellbeing, steps to practising gratitude and so much more: https://greatergood.berkeley.edu/

- Navigate through the Healing Power of ART & ARTISTS (HPAA), an online art gallery "dedicated to raise awareness about how art serves as positive catalyst for enhancing the well-being of individuals, society and the environment": https://www.healing-power-of-art.org/
- You can access and visit different museums for free around London. You can even look for "museums near me" with the *Visit London app*. To know more about it just visit https://www.visitlondon.com/things-to-do/sightseeing/london-attraction/museum/free-museums-in-london
- https://www.nhs.uk/every-mind-matters/. https://www.hee.nhs.uk/sites/default/files/documents/Selfcare%20Handbook%20v3.pdf
- Student nurse healthcare handbook
- https://togetherall.com/en-gb/. This is a 24-hour online community where you can receive support anonymously
- https://www.all4maternity.com/why-does-self-care-matter-for-midwives/. This focusses on self-care specifically for midwives, but maybe useful for others
- https://www.samaritans.org/. Samaritans are available 24 hours a day for counselling support
- https://www.mind.org.uk/
- Cruse offer support for those dealing with bereavement https://www.cruse.org.uk/.
- Winston's Wish is a group that supports bereaved children, young people, their families and the professionals who support them. Although not directly related to clinical practice this has been added for those that may experience personal loss and also have children that need support. https://www.winstonswish.org/
- Civility Saves Lives – https://www.civilitysaveslives.com/. This outlines the impact that being civil at workplace has on improving safety at work.
- Visit and explore the interactive tool *Atlas of Emotions* developed by Dr Paul Ekman (a well-known and influent American psychologist) and Dalai Lama (the spiritual leader of the Tibetan people) where emotions have been divided into major five categories: http://atlasofemotions.org/#introduction/. If you are curious want to know more about the project development and research findings, check The *Atlas of Emotions* with Dr Paul Ekman and Dr Eve Ekman in the University of California Television (UCTV) YouTube channel: https://www.youtube.com/watch?v=AaDzUFL9CLE
- The emotional agility quiz "gives you personalised feedback on how to be more effective with your thoughts and emotions, so you can come to your everyday choices and your life with more intention and insight". Developed by Susan David, a Harvard Medical School psychologist is available here: http://quiz.susandavid.com/s3/eai
- Daniel Goleman podcast series entitled *First Person Plural: EI & Beyond* brings different stories, narratives and theory discussions on emotional intelligence. You can choose from the different episodes here: https://www.keystepmedia.com/first-person-plural/

- The Institute for Health and Human Potential (IHHP) offers a free online resource centre with several emotional intelligence tools: https://www.ihhp.com/resource-center/
- On the Emotional Logic Centre website, you can find developmental tools to improve emotional intelligence. While some of the resources and short courses are not free, you can find free interesting and illustrating videos: https://www.emotionallogiccentre.org.uk/
- Yale Center for Emotional Intelligence (YCEI) offers some free courses on emotional intelligence through Coursera platform. In addition, has a section with up-to-date publications by topic: https://ycei.org/
- IHHP offers a free online resource centre with several emotional intelligence tools: https://www.ihhp.com/resource-center/
- You can explore the tools, activities and resources in the Positive Psychology website and download for free three emotional exercises pack for training emotional intelligence skills. https://positivepsychology.com/emotional-intelligence-exercises/
- Chartered Institute of Personnel and Development (CIPD) Stress in the workplace. https://www.cipd.co.uk/knowledge/culture/well-being/stress-factsheet
- NHS Employers How are you feeling NHS Emotional Wellbeing Toolkit. https://www.nhsemployers.org/howareyoufeelingnhs

Resources

- National Institute of Health. (2021). Physical wellness toolkit. https://www.nih.gov/health-information/physical-wellness-toolkit#:~:text=6%20strategies%20for%20improving%20your%20physical%20health%201,healthy%20diet.%20...%206%20Build%20healthy%20habits.%20
- NHS. (2021). Exercise. https://www.nhs.uk/live-well/exercise/
- Department of Health. (2020). Health matters: physical activity – prevention and management of long-term conditions. https://www.gov.uk/government/publications/health-matters-physical-activity/health-matters-physical-activity-prevention-and-management-of-long-term-conditions
- WHO. (2021). Physical activity. https://www.who.int/health-topics/physical-activity#tab=tab_1
- Public Health England. (2021). Couch to 5K. https://www.gov.uk/government/news/couch-to-5k-app-hits-5-million-downloads
- Digital weight management programme for NHS staff – https://staff.wmp.nhs.uk/
- Walking for health – https://www.walkingforhealth.org.uk/
- Ramblers – https://www.ramblers.org.uk/go-walking
- Meet up – https://www.meetup.com/

- NHS Alcohol units – https://www.nhs.uk/live-well/alcohol-advice/calculating-alcohol-units/
- Alcohol use disorders identification test (AUDIT) – https://assets.publishing.service.gov.uk/government/uploads/system/uploads/attachment_data/file/684823/Alcohol_use_disorders_identification_test__AUDIT_.pdf
- Alcohol use disorders identification test – consumption (AUDIT C) – https://assets.publishing.service.gov.uk/government/uploads/system/uploads/attachment_data/file/684826/Alcohol_use_disorders_identification_test_for_consumption__AUDIT_C_.pdf
- NHS Alcohol Support – https://www.nhs.uk/live-well/alcohol-advice/alcohol-support/
- NHS Local Support – https://www.nhs.uk/nhs-services/find-alcohol-addiction-support-services/
- Talking therapies and counselling – https://www.nhs.uk/mental-health/talking-therapies-medicine-treatments/talking-therapies-and-counselling/benefits-of-talking-therapies/
- NHS Health Risk of smoking – https://www.nhs.uk/common-health-questions/lifestyle/what-are-the-health-risks-of-smoking/
- NICE. (2021). Chronic obstructive pulmonary disease in adults. https://www.nice.org.uk/guidance/qs10/chapter/introduction
- NHS Quit Support – https://www.nhs.uk/better-health/quit-smoking/
- British Nutrition Foundation – Vitamins and Minerals. https://www.nutrition.org.uk/healthy-sustainable-diets/vitamins-and-minerals/. https://www.nutrition.org.uk/healthy-sustainable-diets/vitamins-and-minerals/?level=Consumer
- NHS Eat well. https://www.nhs.uk/live-well/eat-well/
- Very Well fit – Macronutrients 101. https://www.verywellfit.com/macronutrients-2242006
- Puri, N. (2022). Benefits of exercise. https://www.bupa.co.uk/health-information/exercise-fitness/benefits-of-exercise
- British Nutrition Foundation. (2022). Health conditions. https://www.nutrition.org.uk/health-conditions/
- British Nutrition Foundation. (2022). Vitamins and minerals. https://www.nutrition.org.uk/healthy-sustainable-diets/vitamins-and-minerals/
- NHS. (2019). Eating a balanced diet. https://www.nhs.uk/live-well/eat-well/how-to-eat-a-balanced-diet/eating-a-balanced-diet/
- British Nutrition Foundation. (2022). Hydration. https://www.nutrition.org.uk/healthy-sustainable-diets/hydration/
- NICE. (2011). Chronic obstructive pulmonary disease in adults. https://www.nice.org.uk/guidance/qs10/chapter/introduction
- (Rowe, 2020).

- NHS. (2021). Quit smoking. https://www.nhs.uk/live-well/quit-smoking/nhs-stop-smoking-services-help-you-quit/
- NHS. (2021). Exercise. https://www.nhs.uk/live-well/exercise/exercise-health-benefits/
- NHS. (2018). NHS stop smoking services help you quit. https://www.nhs.uk/common-health-questions/lifestyle/what-are-the-health-risks-of-smoking/
- (NHS Inform, 2022). Myths. https://www.nhsinform.scot/healthy-living/stopping-smoking/when-you-stop/myths
- Rowe, K. (2020). Dopamine & serotonin: 2 natural ways to stay motivated and happy. https://brainmd.com/blog/dopamine-and-serotonin/#:~:text=Serotonin%20plays%20multiple%20roles%20in%20the%20brain%E2%80%99s%20functioning%2C,survival%20functions%20like%20body%20temperature%20regulation%20and%20breathing
- Mayo Clinic. (2021). Alcohol use: Weighing risks and benefits. https://www.mayoclinic.org/healthy-lifestyle/nutrition-and-healthy-eating/in-depth/alcohol/art-20044551
- NHS. (2021). Alcohol units. https://www.nhs.uk/live-well/alcohol-advice/calculating-alcohol-units/
- NHS. (2018). Alcohol misuse – overview. https://www.nhs.uk/conditions/alcohol-misuse/

Index

Printed in the USA
CPSIA information can be obtained
at www.ICGtesting.com
JSHW050713010624
63940JS00002B/18

9 781529 767391